Aspects of Biomedicine

Progress and Perspectives of Blood Detoxification

Prospective Studies in Science and Technology

ASPECTS OF BIOMEDICINE
Progress and Perspectives of Blood Detoxification

A report prepared for the Commission of the European Communities, Directorate-General for Science. Research and Development, as part of the FAST Programme (Forecasting and Assessment in the Field of Science and Technology)

by
Elvio Mantovani
Walter Marconi
Rosanna Mosti

ASSORENI, ENI Group Research Association, Italy

Frances Pinter (Publishers), London and Dover N.H.
for the Commission of the European Communities

First Published in Great Britain in 1982 by
Frances Pinter (Publishers) Ltd.
5 Dryden St., London WC2E 9NW

ISBN 0 86187 269 X

Published in the United States of America in 1982 by
Frances Pinter (Publishers)
21 Washington St. Dover, N.H.

Library of Congress Cataloguing in Publication Data

Mantovani, E., 1938-
Aspects of Biomedicine.

Bibliography: P.
Includes Index.
1. Hemodialysis. I. Marconi, W., 1930-
II. Mosti, R., 1935- . III. Title. (DNLM:
1. Hemodialysis. 2. Kidney Failure, Chronic-Therapy.
3. Uremia-Therapy. WJ 378 M293a)
RC901.7.H45M36 1982 617'.461059 82-12345

ISBN 0-86187-269-X

Publication arrangements by
Commission of the European Communities
Directorate-General Information Market and Innovation
Luxembourg

EUR 8059

Printed by SRP, Exeter

TABLE OF CONTENTS

PREFACE

The FAST Programme (Forecasting and Assessment in Science and Technology) was established by decision of the Council of Ministers of the European Community, in July 1978. Its mandate requires it to contribute to the definition of long-term research and development objectives, and to the development of a coherent science and technology policy, for the community, taking account of long-term technical, structural and social change.

The Bio-society sub-programme of FAST focusses on these objectives in the context of recent and long-term potential developments in the applications of the life sciences. It comprises 12 study projects or working group activities. This report describes the results and recommendations of a study financed 70% by the Italian ENI Group of companies 30% by European Community funds.

Biomedical technology is a leading edge of biotechnology, depending on and advancing our understanding of the complexities of human physiology. Of direct concern to afflicted individuals, the deployment of biomedicine is in aggregate of major significance to the whole society, not least in view of its economic impact: renal dialysis represents a billion-dollar-plus public expense each year in both Western Europe and the United States.

The technology and the management of blood detoxification illustrate points of fundamental significance, ranging from specific technical issues to questions concerning the organization of European research.

In preparing their report, Dr Mantovani and his colleagues have drawn on a wide-ranging survey of the relevant literature, have participated in conferences and conducted interviews, and have collated data from many sources, to give a full picture of the situation of renal dialysis in Europe as at 1980/81. The need, the alternative technologies, and the wider social and economic aspects are described. Renal dialysis is a typical example of a halfway technology: expensive and less than fully satisfactory. The current dialysis technologies can be improved on, their costs reduced. The importance of European-scale cooperation and organization is illustrated by the fact that kidney transplantation success rates are already significantly higher in Europe than in the U.S. by virtue of the better tissue matching which the coordinated information and transfer system makes possible. There is scope for further improvement in these success rates: through technical developments, through improvements in cooperation and management, and most immediately through the responsible education of public attitudes to influence the supply of transplantable organs. In the long term, the goal of an implantable, artificial kidney is conceivable.

Complementary to the discussion of renal dialysis is the review of the other potential therapeutic uses of haemapheresis: which are shown to be considerable.

The report describes the commercial structure of the market for dialysis equipment. In the long-established renal dialysis market, the European position is strong. In the newer and higher technology of haemapheresis, it is less so, and there is strong and increasing US and Japanese pressure.

In conclusion, the authors make many practical recommendations for improving treatment modalities and reducing the cost of uremic therapy, emphasising organizational aspects (requiring European coordination) as well as technological improvements. Research targets are:

1. Kidney harvesting and preservation
2. Tissue typing and matching
3. Better immunosuppressive therapies

The need for European cooperation is further stressed in the context of the relatively new and uncertain field of plasmapheresis, in which research will be long-term, expensive and sometimes high risk, requiring public involvement as in the USA. The European research is 'too diversified, dispersed, little coordinated, and the authors conclude that' it is obvious that each European country alone cannot compete with USA and Japan'. They therefore advocate joint community action in order to:

- mobilize competences and potentials
- coordinate activities
- support sectoral policies of the commission

FAST

I. TERMS OF REFERENCE PROVIDED BY THE COMMISSION

The FAST programme is intended to contribute to the definition of long-term Community research and development objectives and priorities, and the sub-programme "Bio-Society" is concerned with those fields in the life sciences which may affect the quality of human life.

The choice of blood detoxification, as object of this study, was suggested by the staggering economic cost supported by the social security systems of the various european countries (around 1000-1200 million U.S. dollars in West Europe in 1981) for the treatment of uremia by dialysis (the most known type of blood detoxification), as well as by the social problems posed by the disabling diseases treated with this therapeutic modality.

Recent applications of various procedures of blood detoxification have suggested that this technique could be effective also in the treatment of a large spectrum of diseases, ranging from certain types of cancer to nervous disorders, and a better definition of such potentialities would be worthwhile.

Moreover, the European market for equipment used in the blood detoxification field is now (1981) worth over 400 million U.S. dollars, and increasing rapidly, so that a strong european industry in this field is desirable.

II. METHODOLOGY OF THE REPORT

This report is intended both for the specialist and the non-specialist, and in consideration of the complexity and variety of the disciplines involved, it will give a general overview of the subject, without being too specific in scientific detail.

The information reported has been collected through literature search (direct and through Medline Data Base) and by participation in meetings organized by various associations active in the field.

Supplementary information has been obtained by personal interviews with a variety of people in, for example, hospitals, research centres, government bodies, non-profit organizations dedicated to health care, distributors, marketing operators, etc. Most of the personal contacts have taken place in Italy, Great Britain, Sweden, and Belgium.

For the purpose of a comparative evaluation, in some cases the situation in the U.S.A. has been taken into account.

III. IDENTIFICATION OF THE SOURCES

Blood detoxification is part of a more general scientific, technological and commercial frame, sometimes generically indicated as biomedicine. Most of the people involved, in one way or another, in this area are associated through organizations, which generally meet once a year, and a careful survey of the proceedings of such meetings has helped very much in the preparation of this report.

In particular we have surveyed the work of four organizations: the American Society for Artificial Internal Organs (ASAIO), the European Dialysis and Transplantation Association (EDTA), the International Society for Artificial Organs (ISAO), and the European Society for Artificial Organs (ESAO). The members of these organizations are scientists essentially from West Europe, U.S.A. and Japan, and their research activities cover various fields of biomedicine as can be seen in Figure 1, where the subjects of the communications presented at the most recent meetings are summarised.

The ASAIO and the EDTA were the first two of these organisations to be formed. The former was established in the mid 1950's, and amongst its over 1200 members are scientists of various disciplines (physicians, chemical engineers, physicists, chemists, surgeons, etc.). In fact, one of its aims is to tackle the problems of biomedicine by a multidisciplinary effort, in order to have a more integral and deeper insight.

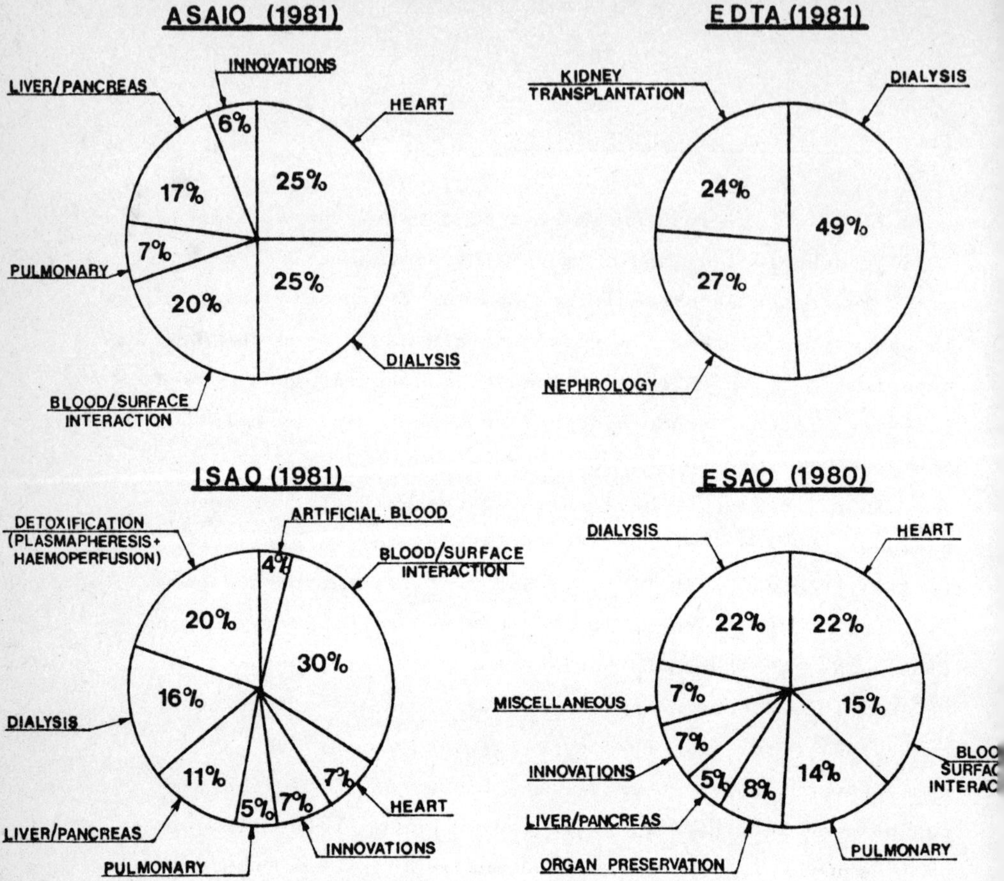

Figure 1 - Breakdown of the fields of research in biomedicine as shown by the Proceedings of the latest meeting held, by the Associations indicated, before 31st July 1981.

EDTA was founded in the early 1960's, and now has about 3000 members, mostly surgeons and nephrologists. The communications presented at its meetings cover essentially the medical side of the problems investigated. Other aims of this association are the collection of statistical data about the patients on treatment for end-stage renal disease and about the centres treating these patients. These figures are very useful both for the specialists and the industry.

The other two associations, ISAO and ESAO, were founded in the mid 1970's and their composition and aims are similar to those of ASAIO.

Attention has been given also to the proceedings of the Congresses of the International Society of Nephrology.

The literature search through Medline Data Base was carried out using key words, covering both the names of the diseases and of selected authors, while the following journals have been surveyed systematically:

- Kidney International
- Nephron
- Clinical Nephrology
- Nouvelle Presse Medicale
- Lancet
- New England Journal of Medicine
- Blood
- Artificial Organs.

Attention has been given also to:

- Dialysis and Transplantation
- Contemporary Dialysis

The International Journal of Artificial Organs has proved particularly helpful for obtaining a general overview of the field because of its multidisciplinary format.

IV. DIALYTIC THERAPY FOR END STAGE RENAL DISEASE

Introduction

In Europe more than 160.000 patients with various diseases of the kidney and urinary tract, various systemic diseases, drug damage etc., which result in renal shut down, die each year from terminal renal failure.

Figure 2 gives the geographical distribution in the majority of European countries of deaths related to kidney-urinary tract disorders, together with those reported in the United States and Japan. In Figure 3 this information is restated as the annual death rate per 100.000 people. It shows that in Europe death rates linked to terminal renal failure are generally higher than in the United States and Japan. These death rates, which do vary from country to country, would be even higher if maintenance dialysis were not used routinely.

Renal shut down results in the retention in the patient's blood of urea and other metabolic end products normally excreted into the urine. Dialysis reduces blood water levels and restores solute concentrations, that can no longer be achieved by the natural organ.

This therapeutic technique, however, does not restore the kidney function, since the uremic state represents more than failure of renal excretory functions alone. In fact, a host of metabolic and endocrine functions, normally dependent on functioning kidneys, are also impaired by chronic renal failure. These functions are not replaced by the dia-

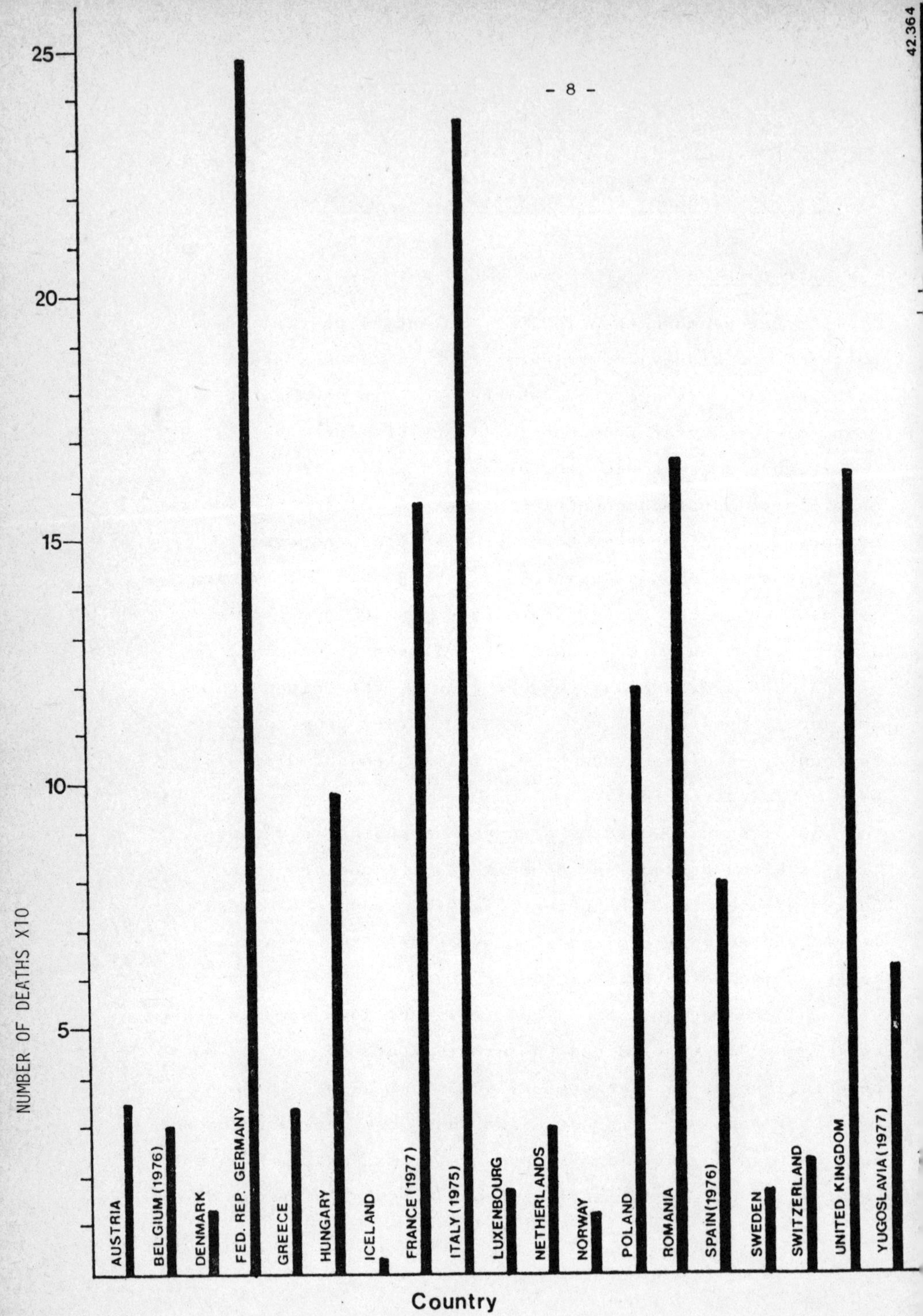

Figure 2 - Total deaths related to kidney-urinary tract disorders in most of Europ
Countries, U.S.A. and Japan. Unless otherwise stated, the data refer to
(The diseases considered are those classified under A105-A111 and A82 b
International Classification of Diseases, 8th Rev. list A).

42.364

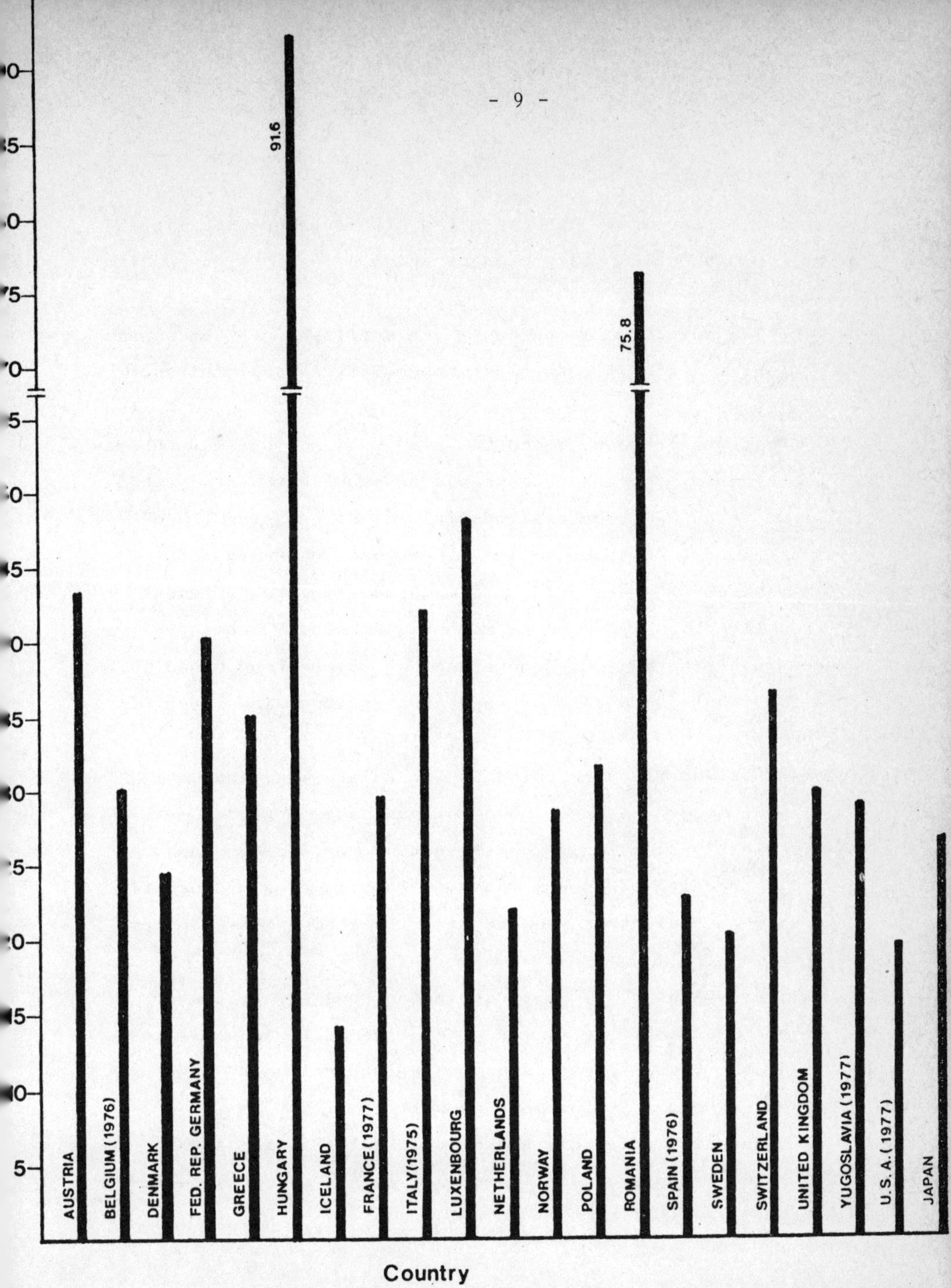

Figure 3 - Number of death per 100,000 people related to kidney-urinary tract disorders. Unless otherwise stated the data refer to 1978. (The diseases considered are those classified under A105-A111 and A82 by International Classification of Disease, 8th Rev. list A).

lytic therapy, nevertheless with this technique the life of the patient can be prolonged and its quality reasonably improved.

Two main procedures have been developed for the management of the dialytic therapy: haemodialysis and peritoneal dialysis.

At the present, haemodialysis is by far the most prevalent therapy for end-stage renal disease. With this method blood which has been treated with an anticoagulant, and a balanced salt solution (dialysate) are perfused to opposite sides of a semipermeable membrane. Solute diffuses from blood to dialysate as a consequence of a concentration gradient. The rate of removal of the solute from blood is a function of membrane surface area and the flow rates of both blood and dialysate. While clearance (molecular removal) is primarily a function of molecular size, and small molecules such as urea and creatinine are extracted more efficiently than larger ones, such as peptide hormones, the extraction of excess water is favored by a hydrostatic pressure gradient from blood to dialysate, across the membrane.

A typical dialysis prescription consists of two or three treatments a week for a total of 12 to 14 or 14 to 18 hours, respectively, and at the present the three times a week schedule is the most popular.

In principle, the equipment used for haemodialysis is rather simple consisting of a machine, which circulates blood and dialysate, and a dialyser, which removes solutes and excess water from blood. The first haemodialysis machines consist of a large tank (200-300 l) in which a concentrated salt solution, containing ions of sodium, calcium, potassium, magnesium, chloride, and either bicarbonate or acetate is diluted. Dialysis is performed until this solution contains too high a concentration of the diffusing solutes. The advantages of such a system are essentially the low cost, simplicity, and reliability, while its disadvantages are bulkiness and poor mobility, possibility of human error in preparing the dialysate, and the considerable operator time necessary to prepare the dialysate.

The second generation machines, are the "proportioning" dialysate-mixing systems. These have simplified dialysate preparation and are particularly suitable for preparing a "personalized" dialysate composition to meet more specifically the needs of the different patients. In the proportioning systems, no solution tank is needed (the dialysate is continuously discarded) and accuracy of dialysate ionic concentration is attained by continuous monitoring of its electrical conductivity. Proportioning systems are relatively small, electronically sophisticated machines. They are rather expensive (12,000-18,000 U.S. dollars), and the newest types use microprocessors for easier operation and control.

To lower the costs of the dialytic therapy, "central" proportioning systems have also been developed, which are used to mix and deliver dialysate for up to 20 dialysis stations. These systems are suitable for out-of-hospital satellite units, where large numbers of stable, chronic patients, not requiring individual dialysate composition, are treated.

One of the problems related to haemodialysis is the large volume of water needed for the conventional procedure of treatment (600 to 700 litres a week). This fact can be a limitation in some cases, and certainly hampers the development of self-contained portable dialysis devices.

Dialysate regeneration can overcome this problem but currently the Redy system (Organon Teknika Inc. Ass., The Netherlands) is the only unit commercially available which makes dialysate regeneration possible, and which has been successfully used for the treatment of many patients (W. Drukker et al., in Replacement of Renal Function by Dialysis, 1978). With this system, dialysate regeneration is achieved by using a cartridge containing urease, which converts urea into ammonia, and charcoal, zirconium oxide, and zirconium phosphate, which adsorb the ammonia and the other solutes in the course of recirculation of a small volume (5.5 litres) of dialysate contained in a reservoir incorporated into the machine.

The efficiency of a dialysis system in removing solute and water from blood, is largely related to the characteristics of the membrane used for the construction of the dialyser.

The great majority of the current disposable dialysers use membranes made with cellulosic material, little different from that used by Kolff in his early experiments (E. Klein, Clin. Nephrol., 1978). However, over the years, considerable improvements in the efficiency of the dialysers have been attained through membrane manufacturing technique, modification of dialyser configuration to provide an even distribution of blood and dialysate, and minimization of the thickness of the blood layer. Nevertheless, cellulosic membranes show a rapid falloff in permeability with increasing molecular weight, especially over 300 daltons, and with the introduction of the "middle molecule" theory (A.L. Babb et al., Trans. ASAIO, 1971 and 1972), membranes with higher cut-off have been sought. In fact, according to this theory, solutes with a molecular weight of 500 to 5000 daltons, still of unknown nature, accumulate in the blood of uremic patients and may cause or contribute to uremic symptoms.

The middle molecule theory has been challenged by many authors (V. Cambi et al., Proc. EDTA, 1972; C.M. Kjellstrand et al., Trans. ASAIO, 1972; R. Maiorca et al., Proc. EDTA, 1974) and supported by many others (J.H. Shinaberger et al., Trans. ASAIO, 1972; N.K. Man et al. Trans. ASAIO, 1973; K.S. Mirahmadi et al., Proc. EDTA, 1974; P.E. Tescham et al., Trans. ASAIO, 1975; H. Asaba et al., Clin. Nephrol., 1979). The question is still unsettled, but nevertheless the middle molecule theory has had a great impact on the design of dialysers, on membrane technology and on dialysis strategies. Non cellulosic membranes, such as those made with polyacrylonitrile and ethylene vinyl alcohol copolymer of higher porosity, have been developed, and dialysers with large membrane area were marketed with the purpose of enhancing middle molecule removal (J. Bergstrom in Replacement of Renal Function by Dialysis, 1978).

Another problem related to the management of haemodialysis is the necessity of having an appropriate vascular access. At present permanent vascular access is attained by internal, arteriovenous fistulas, with venous enlargement for repetitive vein to vein haemodialysis (M.J. Brescia et al., N. Engl. J. Med., 1966). However, external arterio-venous shunts can also be used and they are usually employed in the case of acute renal failure or in the case of difficult vascular access. If a suitable vein is unavailable, and a standard arteriovenous fistula is impractical, a satisfactory alternative can be given by a venous prosthesis in the form of bovine carotid artery or expanded tetrafluoroethylene graft (K.M.H. Butt et al. Curr. Prob. Surg., 1976; L.D. Baker et al., Trans. ASAIO, 1976).

When maintenance dialysis started, one of its main drawbacks was the necessity of blood transfusion to sustain haematocrit (blood count).

Besides the problems posed by the need of quite sizeable quantities of blood, many serious side-effects were associated with that practice: hepatitis, pyrogenic reactions and haemosiderosis were unavoidable with routine transfusion.

With the improvement of the dialytic procedures, however, blood transfusion became generally unnecessary and these problems were lessened; only the recent trend of acceptance of elderly and diabetic patients has brought back the practice of regular transfusion for some patients.

Against blood transfusion was, at first, also the thought that routine blood transfusion could affect adversely subsequent kidney transplantation because it could sensitize the patients and favor rejection.

More recently, however, it has been suggested that blood transfusion could help a subsequent renal transplant (G. Opelz et al., Transplant Proc., 1979).

The phenomenon was not rationalized, but it might be related to the production of "blocking" antibodies, which prevent the attack of the recipient immunologic defenses.

Therefore, it could be worthwile considering a policy of deliberate transfusion, evaluating on the one hand the risk of hepatitis, and on the other the increased success of subsequent renal transplants.

As already mentioned, an alternative to haemodialysis is peritoneal dialysis, which has been little used until very recently, in spite of its relative simplicity compared with haemodialysis.

In this procedure the dialysate is introduced directly into the peritoneal cavity, and blood solute concentration is re-established through exchange, across the peritoneal membrane, between dialysate and the blood flowing in the capillaries of the peritoneal cavity. Because of its ease of initiation (vascular access is not required) peritoneal dialysis is often the procedure of choice when an uremic patient first presents with acute renal failure or with suddenly discovered advanced chronic renal failure. However, peritonitis is a common complication of this technique, and this has been the main reason it has not been widely adopted.

Management of dialysis therapy in Europe

As has already been mentioned, maintenance dialysis has improved the prospects of many patients suffering from renal shut down, and since the first tentative experiments carried out in the early sixties, when dialytic therapy was routinely administered to a small, carefully selected, group of patients (R.M. Hegstrom et al., Trans. Am. Soc. Artif. Intern. Organs, 1961), this technique has evolved dramatically so that about 150.000 patients around the world are now under treatment.

Europe and the United States account each for more than one third of the total and Japan for 21-22 per cent. In these countries the number of patients on maintenance dialysis, is expected to reach a plateau during the next few years and in Figure 4, which reports the increase, of the new patients starting treatment in Europe and some adjacent countries during the period 1972-1979, this trend is evident.

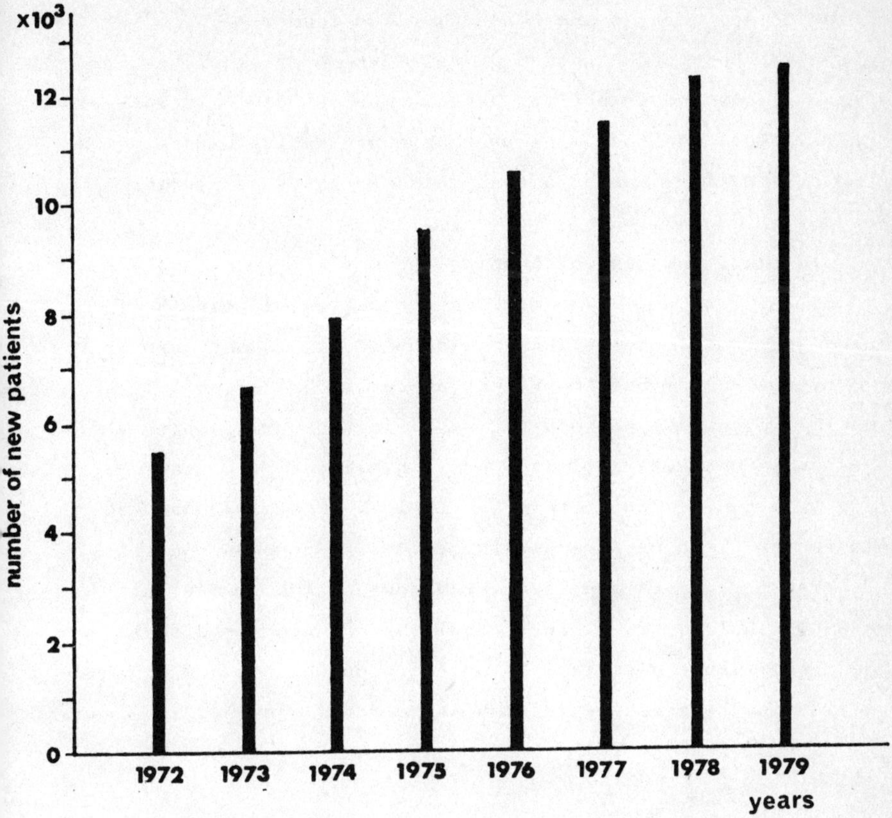

Fig. 4 - Number of new patients starting dialysis in Europe in each of the years, 1972 to 1979. Source : EDTA Registry, 1979.

The present restricted use of dialytic therapy is chiefly due to its huge cost, which puts it beyond the reach of most of the Asian, African and South American countries.

As it has been reported at the 18th Congress of the European Dialysis and Transplant Association (EDTA), held in Paris on July 1981, the countries where the per capita GNP is below 2700 U.S. dollars cannot afford this treatment as routine therapy.

In fact, the cost of hospital haemodialysis is estimated around 25.000-30.000 U.S. dollars per patient a year (E.A. Friedman, Proc. 8th Int. Congr. Nephrol., 1981) and this heavily weights on the budget of the various social security systems which have to foot the bill. In the United States, the total cost will probably pass 2 billion U.S. dollars a year by 1984 (T. Manis et al. N. Engl. J. Med. 1979) and a similar cost can be forecast for the West European countries.

Table 1, gives a partial breakdown of the primary diseases which lead to patients requiring maintenance dialysis. The predominant role played by glomerulonephritis and pyelonephritis in the aetiology of end stage renal disease, is clear.

TABLE 1

Distribution of Primary Diseases in Patients Starting Renal Replacement Therapy in Europe in 1979. (o)

Glomerulonephritis	30.7%
Pyelonephritis/Interstitial N.	21.2%
Multi-system Disease	10.8%
Cystic Kidney Disease	9.2%
Renal Vascular Disease	7.6%
Heredo-familial	2.5%
CRF, Aetiology Uncertain	11.1%
Drug Nephropathy	3.5%
Other	3.4%

(o) Source: EDTA Registry, 1979

Table 2 shows the geographical distribution of primary renal diseases and it is evident that the incidence of the various diseases is not the same in the different European countries.

Sometimes, these variations can be related to differences in diagnostic fashion or in the selection of patients. According to the 1979 EDTA Registry (H. Brynger et al., Proc. 17th Congr. EDTA, 1980), for instance, the distribution of primary renal disease in females aged over 55 years, starting dialysis during 1979 in the Federal Republic of Germany and U.K., shows that pyelonephritis accounted for 40 per cent of the patients in Germany and only 12 per cent in U.K. No patients, over 55 with drug nephropathy were reported in U.K., against 7 per cent in Germany, and since the two countries are rather similar, these differences were explained by differences in selection practice.

Sometimes, on the contrary, the differences probably reflect some geographical factor. The endemic Balkan Nephropathy seems to be one example, since it is found practically only in isolated areas of Bulgaria, Romania and Yugoslavia (P.W. Hall et al., Proc. 8th Int. Congr. Nephrol., 1981).

Geographical factors, should be also responsible for the higher incidence of multi-system diseases, mostly diabetes, among young male patients (15-34 years) in Scandinavia (38%) compared to Italy (3%) (H. Brynger et al., Proc. 17th Congr. EDTA, 1980). In fact, in these two countries there are no big differences in selection practice. The diagnosis of diabetes is straightforward and uniform, and only small differences in the proportion of young patients recorded in these two countries with the diagnosis "chronic renal failure, aetiology uncertain", are observed.

TABLE 2

Geographical distribution of primary renal diseases. Percentage of all patients accepted for treatment in 1979 (and 1974) (o)

PRD	Benelux	Scandinavia	France	Fed.Rep. Germany	Italy	Spain	Switzerland	United Kingdom	Whole registry
CRF,aetiology uncertain	8.8 (1.1)	3.4 (1.0)	11.4 (4.0)	13.4 (1.5)	12.5 (3.5)	19.5 (5.6)	9.8 (1.0)	13.9 (1.9)	11.1 (2.4)
GN*	25.0(40.3)	30.5(36.6)	24.8(35.4)	26.6(39.0)	31.8(55.8)	25.8(49.6	21.1(31.3)	31.1(46.0)	30.7(45.2)
PN/Interstitial N**	15.3(13.7	16.2(19.0)	17.8(17.1)	26.2(29.0)	23.1(17.0)	18.4(16.0)	17.5(20.9)	13.9(17.3)	21.2(19.6)
Drug nephropathy	13.4(11.0)	3.4 (6.9)	1.6 (1.7)	5.0 (4.9)	1.0 (1.0)	0.4 (0.3)	17.5(19.9)	1.2 (1.4)	3.5 (3.5)
Cystic kidney disease	10.1(13.5)	11.6(12.3)	11.7 (9.2)	7.3 (8.5)	7.3 (7.3)	10.0 (6.4)	11.9 (7.0)	12.1(10.0)	9.1 (9.0)
Heredo-fami-lial	3.1 (2.7)	1.5 (3.1)	4.3 (7.2)	1.6 (3.2)	2.3 (1.2)	3.1 (5.6)	0.5 (6.5)	3.1 (3.5)	2.5 (3.5)
Renal vascular disease	8.2 (4.6)	6.1 (4.5)	12.4(11.5)	4.8 (2.8)	8.9 (4.7)	9.9 (8.1)	4.6 (2.5)	14.1 (7.0)	7.6 (5.3)
Multi-system disease	12.4 (4.6)	24.2(11.7)	11.6 (5.9)	12.1 (5.7)	9.2 (2.7)	7.8 (2.5)	11 .3 (5.5)	8.3 (4.8)	10.8 (5.0)
Other	3.8 (8.5)	2.9 (4.8)	4.3 (8.1)	3.0 (5.4)	3.9 (6.8)	4.9 (5.9)	5.7 (5.5)	2.2 (8.2)	3.4 (6.6)

(o) Source:EDTA Registry, 1979.

* Glomerulonephritis

** Pyelonephritis/Interstitial nephritis

Particular attention should be given to the large fluctuation in the proportion of patients with drug nephropathy, which is also probably related to geographical factors.

In fact, the incidence of drug nephropathy ranges from values as low as 0.4, 1.0 per cent, in Spain and Italy, respectively, to 17.5 per cent in Switzerland. An interesting study has been made on this topic (J.L. Vanherweghem, 1981) and it has been observed that in Belgium, where analgesic nephropathy accounts for 18.4 per cent of the total (even higher than in Switzerland), the number of patients with this diagnosis is higher in the region of Antwerp, where the factories producing analgesics are concentrated. This is considered a determining factor, and in effect, in Switzerland, where also the drug nephropathy is very high, there is a high concentration of pharmaceutical factories producing analgesics.

This data suggest that in cases like this an appropriate policy could keep this type of disease under control and in fact the decrease registered in Scandinavia, where "drug nephropathy" dropped from 6.9% in 1974, to 3.4% in 1979, could be related to the restrictions introduced in these countries on the sale of analgesics.

Table 2 shows also that the incidence of the various primary renal diseases in patients starting dialysis has changed significantly since 1974. The increase of "chronic renal failure (CRF), aetiology uncertain" has been explained by the tendency of the doctors to admit their uncertainty, while the drop of more than 10% for "glomerulonephritis" and the increase for "renal vascular disease" and "multi-system disease" has been related to the increase in age of patients admitted to dialysis.

Glomerulonephritis, in fact, is a disease of younger patients, while vascular diseases and multi-system diseases are typical of older patients.

In Figure 5 the age distribution of patients starting hospital haemodialysis in 1975 and 1978 is compared. The tendency to admit older patients is clearly evident, and this trend has continued also during the last two years, so that now the average age of new patients is over 47 years, up from 42 years in 1975.

Table 3 gives the number of centres and the number of patients on treatment, in Europe and some neighbouring countries, on 31 December 1979.

It can be seen that the number of patients on treatment has grown to over 40,000, however the actual figure was certainly around 50,000, because in some countries many centres have not replied to the EDTA. In Italy, for instance, where only 198 centres out of 284 have replied, the total number of patients on treatment on December 1979 was 11,289, or 199.1 per million polulation, as recorded by the Italian Association for Hemodialysed Patients (ANED), which traced down all centres. Detailed figures for the situation on 1981 were not available, but it is estimated that at present the number of patients on treatment is close to 60,000.

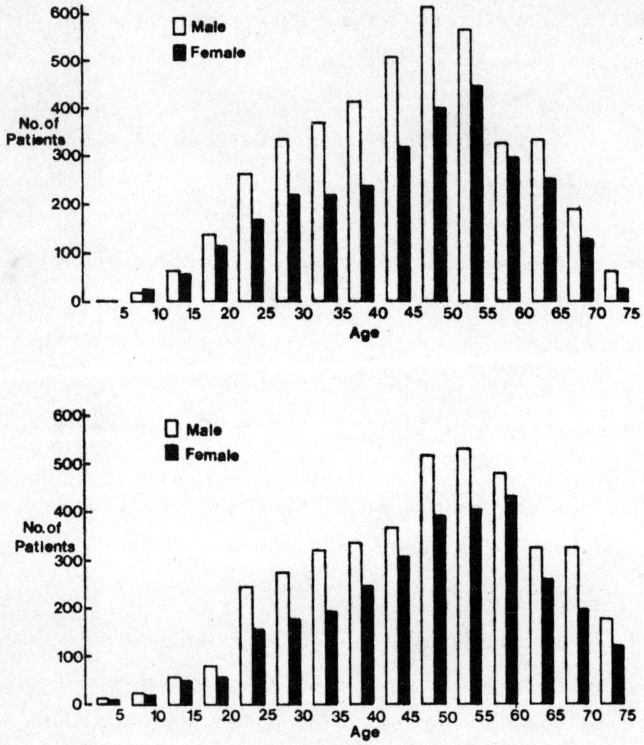

Figure 5 - Age at start of hospital haemodialysis patients on 1975 (top), and 1978 (bottom).
Source: EDTA Registry, 1978 .

TABLE 3

Summary of centres and numbers of patients on treatment on 31st December, 1979

Country	Pop. in mill.	CENTRES Known	CENTRES per mill. pop.	CENTRES Replied	PATIENTS ON TREATMENT AT 31st DECEMBER, 1979: On PD Hosp.	On PD Home	On haemodialysis/ haemofiltration Hosp.	On haemodialysis/ haemofiltration Home	Total	% Home of total	Per mill. pop.
Austria	7.5	19	2.5	19	0	3	640	46	686	6.7	91.5
Belgium	9.8	52	5.3	44	13	45	1.214	98	1.312	7.5	133,9
Bulgaria	8.8	8	0.9	7	0	0	172	0	172	0	19.6
Cyprus	0.6	2	1.6	2	0	0	3	0	3	0	5.0
Czechoslovakia	15.2	18	1.2	17	0	7	421	1	422	0.2	27.8
Denmark	5.1	12	2.4	11	16	36	294	89	383	23.2	75.1
Egypt	39.6	4	0.1	3	0	0	41	1	42	2.4	1.1
Fed.Rep.Germany	61.3	250	4.1	216	123	38	6,676	1,751	8,427	20.8	137.5
Finland	4.8	21	4.4	21	15	11	150	4	154	2.6	32.1
France	53.3	182	3.4	179	150	295	6,624	1,389	8,013	17.3	150.3
German Dem.Rep.	16.8	44	2.6	43	10	0	622	0	622	0	37.0
Greece	9.3	45	4.8	27	10	0	566	3	569	0.5	61.2
Hungary	10.7	7	0.7	7	2	0	137	0	137	0	12.8
Iceland	0.2	1	4.5	1	0	0	6	0	6	0	30.0
Ireland	3.2	4	1.3	4	2	0	77	38	115	33.0	35.9
Israel	3.7	24	6.5	24	29	24	486	69	555	12.4	150.0
Italy	56.7	284	5.0	198	163	77	6,851	902	7,753	11.6	136.7
Lebanon	3.0	2	0.7	2	0	0	32	0	32	0	10.6
Luxembourg	0.4	4	10.0	4	0	0	49	0	49	0	122.5
Netherlands	13.9	43	3.1	41	5	5	1,194	126	1,320	9.5	95.0
Norway	4.1	17	4.2	16	5	6	114	5	119	4.2	29.0
Poland	35.0	38	1.1	31	32	6	340	0	340	0	9.7
Portugal	9.8	8	0.8	6	1	0	137	1	138	0.7	14.1
Spain	37.1	132	3.6	107	101	24	3,430	231	3,661	6.3	98.7
Sweden	8.3	28	3.4	28	35	30	417	120	537	22.3	64.7
Switzerland	6.3	32	5.1	31	20	40	642	192	834	23.0	132.4
Tunisia	6.2	3	0.5	3	0	0	50	0	50	0	8.1
Turkey	43.2	11	0.3	9	3	0	82	0	82	0	2.0
United Kingdom	55.9	57	1.0	55	64	132	1,144	2,042	3,186	64.1	57.0
Yugoslavia	21.9	56	2.6	29	5	0	926	0	926	0	42.3
TOTAL	551.7	1,408	2.5	1,185	804	779	33,537	7,108	40,645	17.5	73.8

Source: EDTA Registry, 1979

Table 3 shows also that the number of patients per million population can be very different from one country to another, and the reasons for such differences are not the same in every case. Among the West European Countries, the differences depend largely on the different incidence of kidney transplantation which is rather low in Italy, the Federal Republic of Germany and France and much higher in the rest of West Europe. On the contrary, the low values observed for the other countries reflect a low availability of renal replacement therapy, due to economic restraints and/or poor medical practice. In fact, the organization of a network of dialysis centres is costly, and requires a health and social security system of high standard.

In Europe, no governmental regulations exist for acceptance into uremia therapy and all patients requiring this therapy are supposed to be treated. In effect, this seems to be true in many European countries, such as Italy, France, Switzerland, the Federal Republic of Germany and Belgium, where also high risk patients are treated. However, in other countries, notably the U.K., there are more limitations for acceptance into renal replacement therapy. In the former countries, for instance, the number of diabetic patients accepted on dialysis has increased steadily during the last years, as the average age of new patients has increased (see figure 5). In the U.K., on the contrary, increasing age is a strongly limiting factor for acceptance on dialysis therapy. This is clearly demonstrated in Figure 6, where the rate of acceptance of new patients, in relation to age, is compared for the four major West European countries.

Table 3 shows also that hospital haemodialysis is by far the most prevalent therapeutic procedure, though sometimes, home dialysis may cover a significant fraction of the total. Home haemodialysis is often favoured because it can better suit the needs of patient and help their rehabilitation, giving them the freedom to choose their therapeutic schedules. However, economic factors also favour home dialysis, since its cost is about half that of hospital treatment. In the U.K., where economic factors are taken strongly into consideration, home dialysis covers a strikingly high 64% of the total. However, it has been pointed out that this 64% is equivalent to 31 patients per million population, which is considered close to the maximum suitable for treatment in this way (H.J. Gurland, Proc. Second Meet. ISAO, 1979). In fact home dialysis, notwithstanding its advantages, has some limitations. Not all homes offer suitable facilities; a partner is not always available to assist the patient; both patient and partner require training in the dialysis procedure; and an efficient supporting organization must be available to cope with emergency situations. These factors all influence the amount of home dialysis which is possible, and it is questionable whether this procedure could ever be applied to more than 30-35 patients per million population, even in countries which favour this type of therapy.

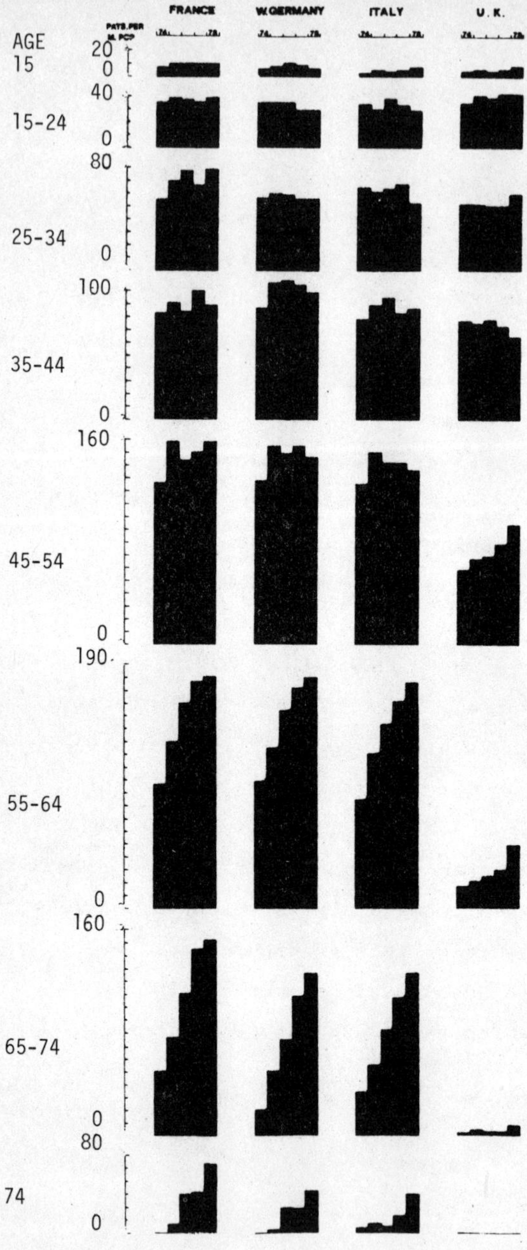

Figure 6 - The rate of acceptance of new dialysis patients (male and female) in relation to population age structure in four countries, 1974-1978.
Source: EDTA Registry, 1979.

Dialysis Strategies

Though the basic principles of dialytic therapy have remained unchanged over the years, many changes in technique have taken place. These changes have involved the machines, the dialysers, the duration of treatment, and the dialytic procedure.

The dialysers, which can be considered the heart of the artificial kidney, have undergone drastic modifications, especially in their design, from the first types used when maintenance dialysis started as routine therapy. The first dialysers were the Kiil type (F. Kiil, Acta Chir. Scand., 1960), later modified by Scribner and colleagues (J.P. Pendras et al., Trans. ASAIO, 1961; J.J. Cole, ibid., 1962). These consist essentially of two sheets of cellulose membrane which separate the dialysate from blood, flowing between the two sheets.

These dialysers, or variants of them, were the most widely used until the late 1960's. However, by 1975 they were applied to only about 14% of European patients(H.J. Gurland et al., Proc. EDTA, 1976). Currently, except in U.K., the use of non-disposable parallel-flow dialysers is coming to an end, and now amounts to less than 4% of the total (EDTA Registry, 1979).

Besides a high (blood) priming volume one of the main limitations of these dialysers is the necessity of resterilization. Formaldehyde is used for this purpose and, when it is incompletely rinsed out, residual traces may give rise to toxic reactions. Residual formaldehyde probably stimulates the N-antibodies which develop in the blood of patients using such equipment.

The majority of dialysers presently used are totally disposable and are of three types: parallel plate, coil and hollow fibers, depending on membrane shape and assembly procedure.

The current disposable flat-plate dialysers use a multilayer design and retain the advantages of the Kiil-type (low flow resistance and a wide range of ultrafiltration), while overcoming many of the objections to their use.

Being fully disposable they are rarely associated with pyrogenic reactions. They are sterilized by γ-rays or ethylene oxide, instead of formaldehyde, and only limited rinsing is necessary before reuse. Their major disadvantage is cost; however, currently, in Europe they are used by about 43% of patients (EDTA Registry, 1979).

Coil dialysers, which are the cheapest disposable type, consist of a tubular membrane, through which the blood flows "normal" to the dialysate. They do have a high flow resistance and require blood pumps for their use but they can be sterilised either by γ-rays or ethylene oxide. Their main advantage is their high ultrafiltration rate, which is beneficial for overhydrated patients.

Hollow fibre dialysers consist of a bundle of hollow fibers, made from regenerated cellulose (Cuprophan) or cellulose acetate. Dialysate flows on the outside of the fibres while blood flows in a countercurrent direction through the fibres, which have an inside diameter of 200 to 300 μm.

The hollow fibre dialysers have a low priming volume, a low compliance and a high surface area to priming volume ratio.

Unlike the first models, the current hollow fibre dialysers may be sterilised by ethylene oxide, and this has certainly helped their diffusion. Their high cost is still one of their main drawbacks, but their good performance has led to their wider acceptance. These dialysers will probably become the most widely used.

Table 4 shows the change in the proportion of different dialysers used between 1974 and 1979, in Western Europe.

TABLE 4

Proportion of patients on hospital and home haemodialysis, in Europe using different dialysers in 1974 and 1979. (o)

Type of dialysers	Per cent of patients	
	1974	1979
Non disposable parallel-flow	20.0	4.0
Disposable parallel-flow	33.5	43.5
Disposable coil	38.5	22.0
Hollow fibres	8.0	30.5

(o) Source: EDTA Registry, 1979.

From Table 4 the changes which occurred between 1974 and 1979 are clearly apparent. There was a spectacular increase in the use of hollow fibre dialysers and a sharp decline in the use of non-disposable parallel-flow and coil dialysers. The reasons for these changes are to be found in the much higher dialysis surface area to priming volume ratio offered by the disposable parallel flow dialysers (especially the newest types, the so called capillary films) and by the hollow fiber dialysers. These models have large dialysis surfaces, which offer higher clearance and higher ultrafiltration rates. As a result of their higher efficiency they have made shorter dialysis schedules possible.

As already pointed out, the number of treatments per week has changed drastically during recent years and while in 1973 almost 70% of patients were treated twice a week for an overall duration of 13-14 hours, at the present almost 90% of patients are treated three times a week for a total of 14-18 hours, whether on home or hospital haemodialysis. However, though the patient feels generally more comfortable on the three times a week schedule, organizational factors tend to determine the timing rather than the patients themselves (H. Brynger et al., Proc. EDTA, 1980).

Not all patients with renal failure react in the same way to dialytic treatment. To help patients cope with some of the problems encountered, new modalities of therapy have been made available during recent years.

TABLE 5

Use of sequential ultrafiltration in countries with more than 500 haemodialysis patients(o)

Country	Number of patients with dialyser reported	Number of patients using sequential ultrafiltrati
German Dem.Rep.	725	246 (33.9%)
Sweden	642	137 (21.3%)
Israel	570	118 (20.7%)
Switzerland	756	126 (16.7%)
Austria	784	122 (15.6%)
Spain	3,325	422 (13.3%)
Netherlands	1,413	148 (10.5%)
United Kingdom	3,873	398 (10.3%)
Fed.Rep.Germany	8,463	733 (8.7%)
Italy	6,670	583 (8.7%)
Yugoslavia	890	73 (8.2%)
Belgium	1,374	84 (6.0%)
France	7,716	251 (3.3%)
Totals	40,163	4,076 (10.0%)

(o) Source: EDTA Registry, 1979.

Some of these have become complementary to regular haemodialysis, while others have become the method of first choice.

Sequential ultrafiltration, haemofiltration and continuous peritoneal dialysis are these new alternatives.

Sequential ultrafiltration has been introduced to overcome hypotension or painful muscle cramping, associated with the removal of large volume of fluid (over 3 liters) from patients who gain excessive weight between dialyses.Bergstrom and others (J. Bergstrom et al., Proc. EDTA, 1976; Bergstrom, Clin. Nephrol. 1978) have developed a technique in which ultrafiltration is performed through a standard membrane without dialysis, by stopping the flow of dialysate through the dialyser. In this way, rapid fluid removal is achieved without inducing hypotension or muscle cramping, and now, ultrafiltration for fluid removal, followed by standard haemodialysis for solute removal, has become a standard procedure in many dialysis units for patients who tolerate fluid removal poorly.

In 1979 in Europe about 10% of all patients used ultrafiltration at least once a month, but it was not adopted to the same extent in all countries, as it can be seen in Table 5.

Haemofiltration has gained a place in the renal replacement therapy programmes, however at present less than 2% of all patients are treated with this method in Europe (Table 6).

TABLE 6

Use of haemofiltration in countries with proportions of patients exceeding the European average (o)

Country	Number of patients with dialysers reported	Number of patients using haemofilters
Luxembourg	51	4 (7.8%)
Greece	482	20 (4.1%)
Czechoslovakia	481	15 (3.1%)
Fed. Rep. Germany	8,463	265 (3.0%)
Belgium	1,374	38 (2.8%)
Yugoslavia	890	18 (2.0%)
Netherlands	1,413	22 (1.7%)
Totals	40,163	513 (1.3%)

(o) Source: EDTA Registry, 1979.

In haemofiltration, a membrane of high porosity removes an ultrafiltrate from perfused blood. The ultrafiltration devices used today employ cellulose or polyacrylonitrile membranes and provide better clearance of larger molecules that can be achieved by haemodialysis. Haemofiltration is reported to be superior to haemodialysis also in the treatment of patients with refractory hypertension or cardiac instability (E. Quellhorst et al., Clin. Nephrol., 1979), and, being more effective in extracting middle molecules, this technique is supported by those in favour of the middle-molecules hypothesis. However, though haemofiltration provides effective advantages in the control of hypertension and comparatively easy control of body water, the initial promise of providing a dramatically more effective mean of treating chronic renal failure, has not been fulfilled. Therefore, it is likely that in the near future haemofiltration will remain a relatively difficult and expensive treatment with no widespread clinical applicability.

Particular attention must be given to peritoneal dialysis which has been known for a long time, but which has been little used so far, because of its major complication, peritonitis.

In 1979, only 3.8% of all patients were treated with this method (H. Brynger et al., Proc. EDTA, 1980). However, the data from the EDTA Registry for 1979 indicate that the total number of patients treated with peritoneal dialysis had increased by 70% between 1978 and 1979.

The increasing success of peritoneal dialysis, depends to a large degree on the development of a permanent safe access to the peritoneal cavity, now obtained with the introduction of the Tenchkoff and Toronto Western Hospital peritoneal permanent catheters. But it has been the introduction of continuous ambulatory peritoneal dialysis (CAPD) which has made this technique particularly promising. (R.P. Popovich, Trans. ASAIO, 1976; D.G. Oreopoulos ibidem, 1978).

This technique is machine-free and is based on the continuous presence in the abdomen of a solution for peritoneal dialysis, which is changed four or five times during the day by the patient. Many socioeconomic and medical advantages are associated with CAPD. The socio-economic advantages are that between exchanges the patients can run their usual activities. Independence of machines and the freedom to travel long distances improve the degree of rehabilitation and adaptation. Moreover, CAPD is cheaper than hospital dialysis and this too is an advantage in view of the necessity to reduce the cost of end stage renal disease therapy.

The medical advantages of CAPD, on the other hand, are an improvement with respect to anemia and hypertension, a relative freedom from dietary restrictions, and an adequate biochemical control without fluctuation. CAPD may also be valuable in the treatment of diabetics with end stage renal disease (insulin can be added to the dialysate) and this is probably one of the reasons for the adoption of this method of therapy with older patients.

Recently a new variant of peritoneal dialysis has been introduced (J.A. Diaz-Busco, Am. Soc. Nephr., 1980).

This techique, called continuous cycling peritoneal dialysis (CCPD), is a combination of intermittent peritoneal dialysis and CAPD. In this approach, the patient uses an automatic machine for an overnight cycling of 6-8 litres of dialysate and at the end of this period leaves 2 litres of it in his abdomen. The advantage of CCPD is that the patient is not required to perform exchanges during the day, and this may decrease the incidence of peritonitis. On the other hand, this technique brings back the machine, and this increases the costs.

In conclusion, the improvements made in the field of peritoneal dialysis have been significant and an increase in the adoption of this technique can be predicted.

At the 18th Congress of the EDTA, held in Paris in July 1981, it was reported that on 31st December 1980, 2.4% of all patients currently on the EDTA Register were being treated by CAPD. The highest treatment rates were in the UK and in Switzerland, where more than 5% of patients were on CAPD. However, the problem of peritonitis, especially for prolonged treatment, is far from being solved, and the wider adoption of this technique must await the solution of this and other problems.

V. COMPLICATIONS OF LONG-TERM DIALYSIS THERAPY

Though dialysis, and in particular, haemodialysis, has been recently labelled as the gold standard therapy for end-stage renal failure (C.M. Kjellstrand, Proc. 8th Int. Congr. Nephrol., 1981), many complications, both medical and surgical, are arising from either inadequate control of uremia, or from the treatment itself.

The survival rate of patients in chronic haemodialysis is no better than that following detection of cancer of the breast or after myocardial infarction.

On 1979 4,586 patients on renal replacement therapy (including kidney transplantation) died in Europe according to the EDTA Registry (H. Brynger et al., Proc. 17th Congr. EDTA, 1980). The death rates from various causes, for patients on hospital haemodialysis and peritoneal dialysis, are recorded in Table 7.

The incidence and type of complications related to maintenance dialysis, have been reviewed in detail in various textbooks (Strategy in Renal Failure, E.A. Friedman, ed., John Wiley and Sons, New York, 1978; Replacement of Renal Function by Dialysis, W. Drukker, F.M. Parson, J.F. Maher eds., Martinus Nijhoff, The Hague, 1978; Uremia - Pathobiology of Patients Treated for 10 Years or More. C. Giordano, E.A. Friedman eds., Wichtig Ed., Milan, 1981).

TABLE 7

Causes of deaths in patients on dialysis, in Western Europe on 1979, according to most relevant causes (o)

Causes of death	Percent of all causes of death	
	Hospital haemo-dialysis	Peritoneal dialysis (First choice)
Myocardial ischemia and infarction	11.2	11.3
Hyperkalaemia	4.4	2.7
Haemorragic pericar-ditis	2.2	0.5
Other causes of cardiac failure	9.6	11.3
Cardiac arrest, cause unknown	10.5	6.5
Hypertensive cardiac failure	5.1	0.5
Cerebro-vascular accident	12.5	14.0
Gastro intestinal haemorrage	2.7	3.2
Pulmonary infection (bacterial)	2.4	4.3
Infection elsewhere	1.1	6.5
Septicaemia	6.6	14.0
Patient refused further treatment	1.2	1.1
Suicide	0.8	0.5
Cachexia	3.9	8.6
Malignant diseases	5.2	2.7
Dementia	2.4	0

(o) Source: EDTA Registry, 1979.

In this report we will review those areas which we consider of particular interest.

Problems related to Uremia

From Table 7 it is clearly evident that cardiovascular diseases, including cardiac failure and hyperkalaemia claim the highest toll, with more than 50% of deaths. Antecedent hypertension related to renal disease, sometimes poorly controlled by dialysis and hypertriglyceridaemia (J. Bagdade et al., J. Lab. Clin. Med., 1976) are considered to be among the main factors involved in accelerated development of arteriosclerosis in chronic dialysis patients (A. Lindner et al., N. Engl. J. Med., 1974; F. Thomas et al., Ann. Surg. 1976). However, the exact cause of cardiovascular deaths remains elusive. The potential causes of the vascular damage are depicted on Figure 7 and, as can be seen, a mixture of metabolic, hormonal, hereditary and environmental factors, as well as changes in the physiological condition of the blood associated with dialysis all enter into the equation.

Another factor which adversely affects the death rate due to cardiovascular disorders is established vascular disease secondary to hypertension. The patients in this conditions do particularly badly. Also the mortality rate for patients with diabetes is many times that experienced by non diabetic dialysis patients (F.P. Brunner et al., Proc. EDTA, 1978).

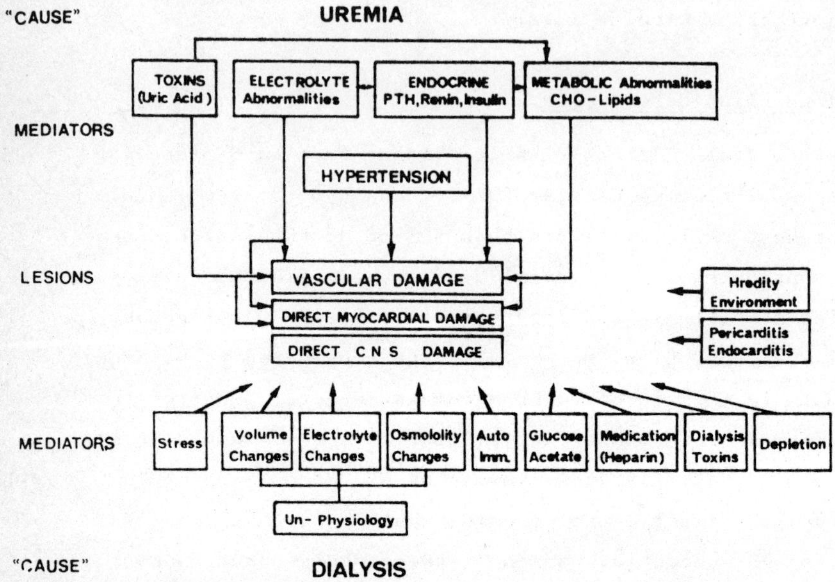

Figure 7 - Possible causes of vascular damage in patients on chronic dialysis.
Either the dialysis procedure or uremia alone can induce vascular damage through all of the mechanisms.
Source: Trans. ASAIO, 1979, p.520.

Ascites are another complication frequently seen in patients on long-term dialysis, usually occurring in catabolic patients (S. Singh et al., Nephron, 1974; L. Gotloib et al., Am. J. Med., 1976). Many hypotheses have been put forward to explain the onset of dialysis ascites, but the problem remains unresolved, and the search for a treatable cause continues.

End-stage renal disease is associated also with endocrine disturbances, which can involve the metabolism of pituitary-gonadal hormones, the thyroid function, adrenocortical hormones, etc.. Sometimes these abnormalities lead to recognizable endocrinopathies (J.P. Knochel, in Replacement of Renal Function by Dialysis, 1978).

Problems related to treatment

Remarkable technological advances have simplified the procedure of haemodialysis and shortened its duration. In spite of this, dialysis remains an unpleasant therapy for the patient, althogh many new procedures, such as sequential dialysis-ultrafiltration, haemofiltration and continuous peritoneal dialysis, have relieved the discomfort and/or prolonged survival.

Hypotension, one of the earliest recognised hazards of haemodialysis, remains common, and even after several months of treatment, mild symptoms of hypotension occur every fourth to sixth dialysis (C.M. Kjellstrand, Dial. Transplant., 1980).

Several pathogenetic mechanisms may be responsible for hypotension during haemodialysis.

Infusion of acetate during dialysis has been suggested as one cause of hypotension, and though the question is controversial, it has been reported that substitution of acetate with bicarbonate reduces the hypotensive symptoms (H. Borges et al., Clin. Res., 1979; U. Greafe et al., Ann. Intern.Med., 1978; B. Wehle et al. Clin. Nephrol., 1978). Volume reduction through ultrafiltration is another likely cause of hypotension, and sequential ultrafiltration has been developed to reduce this problem, although volume removal alone is not considered the only cause of hypotension (J. Bergstrom et al., Proc. Eur. Dial. Transplant Ass. 1976).

Another possible cause for hypotension is the osmolality fall occurring during haemodialysis; emoploying an increased concentration of sodium ions in the dialysate and short-term use of mannitol can be helpful in reducing its incidence (C. M. Kjellstrand, Dial. Transplant., 1980).

Muscle cramps are another common complication associated with the dialytic treatment, particularly with old patients. They tend to occur about once every eight sessions (S. Shaldon, Proc. 8th Congress Nephrol., 1981). Removal of large quantities of fluid has been held responsible for the problem, and ultrafiltration, followed by dialysis, seems to reduce this particular complication (J. Bergstrom et al., Proc. EDTA, 1976).

More complex, and sometimes more dramatic, are the problems due to nonuremic toxicity and hepatitis.

In fact, while in general most, if not all, systemic manifestations of the uremic syndrome are reduced by maintenance dialysis, new complications have been recognized, particularly with patients treated for long periods.

Derivatives of plasticisers, used to manufacture polyvinyl chloride for blood lines, have been detected in the blood of patients on maintenance dialysis (L.M. Lewis, et al., Clin. Chem., 1978), and have been tentatively associated with an illness that simulates hepatitis (J. Neergaard et al., Nephron, 1975). Formaldehyde, often used to sterilize dialysis blood circuits, may be immediately toxic when absorbed in large amounts. However, it can be hazardous also in very small quantities and formaldehyde has been associated with the formation of antibodies against the blood group substance N of the MN system (K.M. Koch et al., Trans. ASAIO, 1978), and with decreased survival of red cells.

Very recently also sterilization with ethylene oxide, at the present the procedure of choice, has raised some concern since this compound has been suspected to be a cancerogenic agent (American Conference Governmental Industrial Hygienists, 1980).

If confirmed, this finding would create many complications especially in consideration of the widespread use of ethylene oxide as sterilizing agent and the Ministries of Health of various countries, such as Italy, Sweden and the United States, have solicited investigations to clarify the question.

Particularly hazardous can be the intoxication due to trace metals. Copper, aluminium, zinc and nickel have been detected in abnormal concentrations in plasma or tissues of patients on long-term dialysis (A.C. Alfrey et al., Replacement of Renal Function by Dialysis, 1978).

Since all these elements bind to plasma proteins, any traces present in the dialysis solution tend to be taken up by the patient during the dialysis session.

Aluminium intoxication is particularly dangerous since aluminium is considered the principal cause, if probably not the only one, of dementia in dialysed patients (D. Brancaccio et al., in Uremia. Pathobiology of Patients Treated for 10 Years or More, 1981).

Dialysis dementia is a progressive degeneration of the central nervous system and is one of the most frightening complications of chronic haemodialysis. In the United Kingdom it occurs in up to 4% of dialysed patients (I.S. Parkinson et al., Lancet II, 1979) and as can be seen in Table 7 it is not a minor cause of death of patients on haemodialysis (no deaths related to this illness are recorded for patients on peritoneal dialysis).

The treatment of the water for the preparation of the dialysate with reverse osmosis and ion exchange resins to eliminate aluminium and other trace metals, is strongly recommended, and a content of aluminium above 50 μg/l should be considered dangerous, since it has been found that this illness occurs more frequently in patients dialysed with unprocessed and softened water (J.S. Parkinson et al., Lancet I, 1979). However, in spite of the universal usage of aluminum-containing antiacids, dialysis dementia has an uneven, peculiar, geographic distribution (A.J. Wing et al., Lancet II, 1980), suggesting that other factors also contribute to this syndrome. Certain medications such as methicillin and narcotics, phosphate depletion, hyperparathyroidism, have been incriminated (L. Taclob et al., Lancet II, 1976; A.M. Pierides et al., Lancet II, 1976; J.H. Ball et al., Nephron, 1977). In all probability, the syndrome involves more than one factor.

The tragedy of this illness has also brought under close scrutiny all procedures which could favour the release of aluminium during the dialytic treatment.

The Redy system, for instance, which uses a cartridge containing aluminum oxide for the regeneration of dialysate, has raised some doubts about its prolonged use, since the release of aluminium can be foreseen, especially when bicarbonate is present in the dialysate (B. Branger et al., Proc. EDTA, 1980).

The complexity of social and medical problems related to aluminium intoxication has prompted the Registry of the European Dialysis and Transplantation Association (EDTA) to mount an inquiry into the extent of dialysis dementia in Europe (A.J. Wing et al., Lancet II, 1980), and more recently also the European Economic Community has launched

(Directorate General V, September 1981) an investigation for the definition of quality requirements of water used for the preparation of dialysate.

Renal osteodystrophy is another illness which is particularly serious in uremic patients and seems to be worsened by regular haemodialysis (bone diseases are very limited in patients on peritoneal dialysis). The mechanism linking haemodialysis and bone disease has not been identified with certainty but various conditions related to this therapy, which may affect bone structure and metabolism, have been pin-pointed (J.W. Coburn, in Replacement of Renal Function by Dialysis, 1978). These include the use of heparin, as an anticoagulant, the calcium and magnesium content of dialysate, impurities of water and the use of fluorinated water for the preparation of dialysate. Moreover, during long-term therapy with haemodialysis, the blood level of parathyroid hormone was found to increase (S.G. Massry et al., in Uremia. Pathobiology of Patients treated for 10 Years or More, 1981). A correlation between the duration of haemodialysis and hyperparathyroid bone disease has been suggested, probably due to intermittent or persistent hyperphosphatemia (E. Slatopolsky et al., in Vitamine D. Basic Research and its Clinical Applications, 1979).

Since the early days of maintenance dialysis, hepatitis B has been a serious threat both to the patients and staff of dialysis units. At the present the reduced frequency of transfusions, the availability of a radioimmunoassay to detect hepatitis B surface antigen (HBsAg), which permits detection and isolation of patients carrying this virus, and sanitation measures such as the use of hepatitis B immunoglobulin (HBIG), have lessened the hazard due to this virus (D.R. Snidman et al., Ann. Intern. Med., 1975; A.M. Prince et al., J. Infect. Dis., 1978). However, the problem of hepatitis B has not been eliminated, and in some centres its incidence is still too high. Recently, a vaccine against hepatitis B has been developed and controlled clinical trials have demonstrated its efficacy (W. Szmuness et al., Lancet II, 1980; J. Crosnier et al., Lancet II, 1981; J. Crosniet et al., 1981), so that there are many hopes that this problem could eventually be overcome. However, in recent years an increasing number of patients became ill for non A - non B hepatitis, whose origin is still controversial (P. Coursaget et al., Nouv. Presse Med., 1978; M.M. Avram. Proc. 16th Meeting EDTA, 1979; R.M. Galbraith et al.,Lancet, 1979; J.P. Mery et al., Nouv. Press Med., 1979). During the 1980 EDTA Meeting, the danger of non A - non B hepatitis was stressed, and it was reported that in the Federal Republic of Germany and France almost 20% of all centres reported cases of non A - non B hepatitis (H. Brynger et al., Proc. 17th EDTA Meeting, 1980). Considering that in the Netherlands, Sweden and the United Kingdom more cases of non A - non B hepatitis than hepatitis B are reported, an aggressive effort should be made to tackle this problem.

Different kinds of complication are posed by peritoneal dialysis, which, as already pointed out, seems to lessen some of the problems associated with the dialytic therapy. As can be seen from Table 7, this treatment method leads to a reduced death rate from cardiovascular disorders, and seems to eliminate deaths due to dementia.On the other hand, the higher rate of deaths due to infections is evident and in fact peritonitis has been always the major problem associated with peritoneal dialysis, hampering also the diffusion of continuous peritoneal dialysis (CAPD and CCPD). A safe permanent access to the peritoneal cavity is still the problem. Recently a new model, which eliminates the surgical replacement of the catheter, a problem with both the Tenckoff and the Toronto Western Hospital catheters, has been proposed (R. Cavagna, Int. J. Artif. Organs, 1981). Another problem, which is particularly relevant with continuous peritoneal dialysis, is that as a conseguence of the continuous presence of dialysate in the peritoneal cavity, a loss of 6 to 10 grams of protein a day is suffered by the patient (R. Khanna, Periton. Dial. Bull., 1981). The loss of proteins, including albumin, is higher if peritonitis occurs (M.J. Blumenkrantz, Kidney Internat., 1981), and the patients on peritoneal dialysis can develop progressive malnutrition and waste, which can lead to higher death rates from cachexia (Table 7).

The dietary regime of the patient is a very important factor in lessening the hazards associated with the dialytic therapy. In fact, malnutrition and wasting are common in patients on maintenance dialysis (V. Richards et al., Kidney Internat., 1978; G. Guarnieri et al., Am. J. Clin. Nutr., 1980), and an appropriate diet has proved to be helpful for the wellbeing of the patient. A low protein diet has led to increased survival rates (C. Giordano, in Uremia, Pathobiology of Patients Treated for 10 Years or More, 1981), and a supplement of essential amino acids, coupled with a reduced phosphate intake, have improved the efficacy of this dietary regime (H.A. Lee et al., Nutr. Metab., 1980). More recently, the advent of keto-acid analogues of certain amino acids has been considered to represent an improvement in the treatment of chronic renal failure, not only because they make a near protein free diet possible, but also because such a dietary regime involves a reduced intake of potassium and hydrogen ions, and less risk of producing toxic nitrogenous metabolites. The ketoacids therapy has been strongly supported by some (A. Heidland et al., Am. J. Clin. Nutr., 1978) and challenged by others (H.A. Lee et al. in Uremia - Pathobiology of Patients Treated for 10 Years or More, 1981), and its value is still unsettled.

VI. SOCIO-ECONOMIC PROBLEMS ASSOCIATED WITH MAINTENANCE DIALYSIS

As already pointed out at the beginning of this report, maintenance dialysis which, on the one hand has the great merit of allowing the survival of patients who would otherwise die because of insufficient renal function, on the other hand poses serious socio-economic problems. These are due mostly to the cost of the treatment and the need to rehabilitate the patients.

With an average cost estimated at 130-160 U.S. dollars per treatment, it is easy to see the impact on the budget of the public health institutions responsible for the management of this therapy, if one considers that in 1981 there are in Europe more than 55.000 patients on treatment, most of whom are treated three times a week.

It has been reported (E. Friedman, Proc. 8th Int. Cong. Nephrol., 1981) that in the United States the End-Stage Renal Disease Program, with only 0.2% of all patients, consumes 5% (more than 1 billion dollars), of the total Medicare budget. It is pointed out that there is increasing pressure to reduce the expenses absorbed by renal replacement therapy. In this respect, at least in the United States, one of the ways suggested to fight the increase of the costs is to bring back home dialysis which in recent years has been less used although its cost is about a half of that of hospital haemodialysis. The recent advances in peritoneal dialysis probably favour its increased use, but, as already pointed out in this report, it is believed that home dialysis cannot be expanded beyond a certain level, since specific conditions are necessary if a patient is to be treated at home.

Moreover, the apparently lower cost of home dialysis is somewhat misleading. True, the cost of the staff, certainly very high in hospital, is avoided, but in calculating the actual cost of home dialysis, one should also take into account the cost of providing a partner, most often the spouse or a relative, as well as the cost of energy, water, etc. These additional expenses are usually met by the patient himself.

In Europe, the United Kingdom has the highest number of patients on home dialysis (64% on 1979), and in this country the number of patients on maintenance dialysis is also kept down both by strict selection rules, which tend to exclude high risk patients (old people, diabetics etc.), and by favouring kidney transplantation.

However too strict selection rules pose serious ethical problems to the physicians since acceptance on treatment or not, can mean the difference between life and death.

In some countries another way to fight the costs has been the creation of out of hospital satellite units, which need only the equipment for dialysis and staff for assistance. New computer controlled equipment can favour the wider use of such units. In the United Kingdom, a programme aimed at a further reduction of the cost of satellite units is under development by the Department of Health and Social Security.

This programme uses Minimal Care Dialysis Units (MCDU), and is intended for patients who do not require expensive long-term Hospital Centre dialysis and do not have the facilities for, or the capabilities of, long-term home dialysis. They include single patients, patients with a disabled spouse or helper, patients with no home and patients awaiting early transplantation.

The Minimal Care Dialysis Unit programme foresees a centre with a minimum of trained staff, and a maximum of self care by the patient, who is directly involved in the management of the treatment (the reuse of both dialyser and blood lines is also considered).

In the other West European countries home dialysis is less used, and varies greatly (see Table 3) from one country to another, ranging from around 20% as in France, the Federal Republic of Germany or Switzerland, to around or below 10% as in Italy, Belgium or Sweden. A programme similar to MCDU is under development also in Italy, sponsored by ANED, and we do think that a similar programme, or variants of it, could be effective in reducing costs and would be in some respects superior to home dialysis.

Although the cost of the dialysers, generally an average of 22-25 U.S. dollars for the parallel-plate and hollow fiber dialysers using cellulose membranes (the polyacrylonitrile membranes cost around 60 U.S. dollars), accounts for a relatively low portion of the total cost of each dialysis (15-20%), the reuse of filters can help to keep down the cost of dialytic therapy. In fact, a careful study on the cost effectiveness of multiple dialyzer use, has shown that by an appropriate programme to manage the reuse (not all patients surveyed reused membranes), a net 40% saving on the cost of dialysers can be achieved (D.A. Ogden et al., Dial. Transplan., 1981). However, reuse has various drawbacks (formaldehyde for example, necessary for sterilization, can give allergic reactions) and a number of organizations in the U.S.A., such as the Food and Drug Administration, the Health Industry Manufacturers Association, the National Association of Patients in Haemodialysis and Transplant, have expressed opposition to reuse.

Nevertheless, the need for reducing costs in every possible way, should encourage investigation of factors that affect and effect the safe regeneration of dialysers with intact function. This could be achieved by using appropriate materials, by design and manufacture of dialysers with maximum potential for multiple reuse, as well as by education of patients, staff, and physicians.

In any case, the improvement of available techniques and the introduction of new modalities of treatment, is absolutely necessary, not only if we want reduce the economic impact of this treatment method on the resources available for health care, but also if we want to bring this therapeutic technique within the reach of the poor countries which, at the present, are practically excluded from the benefits associated with it.

Continuous Ambulatory Peritoneal Dialysis (CAPD) seems promising in reducing the costs, and in fact in UK and Switzerland almost 6% of patients were treated with this procedure on 1980 (C. Jacobs et al., Congress EDTA, 1981): however many problems, especially those related to the danger of infection, need to be solved before this technique is more widely used.

Another, not secondary, problem associated with renal replacement therapy, is its impact on the social life of the uremic patient, since uremia is a disabling disease and the life of a patient is often far to be normal. In fact, it must be kept in mind that a patient on dialysis is not a healthy person since this therapy overcomes only some aspects of his illness, so that only a certain number of patients are rehabilitated to a degree which allows them to work.

In Europe, in 1979, over 80% of patients on home dialysis, and around 60% on hospital dialysis were thought able to work (Brynger H., et al., Proc. EDTA, 1980). However, only a limited number of these patients do, in fact, find a job.

In 1975, amongst those classified as able to work, only around 35% of hospital dialysis patients were working full time (H.J. Gurland et al., Replacement of Renal Function by Dialysis, 1978). Unfortunately we do not have more recent figures, but at present, the proportion of patients working full time is unlikely to be much higher. As a consequence of that, public programmes to support uremic patients are necessary and in many European countries economic support is provided to the patients that cannot work.

Besides the problems related to the possibility of working, other factors are influencing the "quality of life" of the patients on end-stage renal therapy. Various criteria can be adopted to define the quality of life, but in general "good" quality of life includes:

- ability to adapt to a life with dialysis;
- maintaining and resumption of social contacts and activities which the patient had prior to the illness;
- to work either full or part-time in competitive gainful employment, or with work at home, or studies;
- no or insignificant reduction in standard of living.

However, these goals are not easy to attain because the stresses of dialysis produce anxiety, depression, sexual problems, uncooperativeness and psychosis, which all affect rehabilitation and sometimes lead to suicide. One of the main problems with haemodialysis is the restriction of freedom due to the frequent treatment sessions and the sense of being bound to a technically complicated machine.

In this respect, an improvement has been obtained with the new treatment modalities, notably continuous peritoneal dialysis (CAPD, CCPD), but certainly psychological problems and personality factors play a fundamental role in determining patient rehabilitation.

Women, for example, are generally rated as having a much better life adjustment than men. It is thought that this is partly explained by the fact that society places greater demands upon men to be productive at outside work, while the performance of household activities, with its more flexible demands, is a more feasible goal.

In conclusion, rehabilitation of patients on renal replacement therapy is a very important problem, both economically and socially, and in view of the many factors influencing its success, rehabilitation should start earlier, perhaps even before the patient has actually been started on a dialysis programme.

VII. KIDNEY TRANSPLANTATION

As already mentioned, maintenance dialysis does not restore the kidney function in uremic patients and cannot be performed indefinitely. Therefore, this report cannot leave aside kidney transplantation which is, at the present, the only way to restore the kidney function and bring back the patient to a reasonably normal life.

The 1979 EDTA Registry has reported that on 31st December 1979, in addition to 40,645 patients on haemodialysis /haemofiltration, there were 10,287 patients with a functioning transplant (H. Brynger, Proc. EDTA, 1980), and this number is going to increase since one of the goals of maintenance dialysis should be to keep the patient alive long enough to permit kidney transplantation.

Unfortunately, the small number of suitable organs available each year is the governing factor which limits the application of this treatment modality.

Kidneys for transplantation can be obtained either from living donors or cadavers, however the success of a graft depends heavily on the matching of the transplanted organ with the recipient.

Favourable matching is more probable between relatives and in effect, the highest probability of success is expected when the transplant is performed between monozygote twins.

TABLE 8

Transplantation Rates in European Countries, 1979 (o)

COUNTRY	TRANSPLANTATION RATE PER MILL. POP.		
	CAD	LD	ALL*
Finland	22.9	1.7	25.6
Sweden	14.9	5.2	21.3
Norway	12.9	6.3	20.7
Denmark	17.6	0.6	19.8
Belgium	17.2	0.8	19.2
Ireland	11.9	3.8	16.3
United Kingdom	11.6	1.7	15.1
Switzerland+	11.9	0.2	14.4
Israel	10.0	2.2	13.0
Cyprus	0	10.0	11.7
Iceland	10.0	0	10.0
Austria	8.7	0.3	9.6
Netherlands	7.1	0.2	9.4
France	5.1	0.2	7.1
German Dem. Rep.	6.3	0	6.4
Fed. Rep. Germany	5.3	0.1	6.1
TOTAL EDTA REGISTRY	4.6	0.6	6.0
Spain	2.9	0.7	3.9
Greece	0.5	2.4	2.9
Italy	1.9	0.3	2.7
Hungary	2.0	0.3	2.3
Yugoslavia	0.5	0.5	1.1

* Includes grafts where donor was not stated

\+ Data incomplete.

(o) Source: UK Transplant Service, Annual Report 1980.

However, the number of parents, children, and siblings of uremic patients is limited by nature and is further diminished by the extent of human willingness to donate one of a pair of essential organs. Thus, transplant effort and its future expansion depend on increased availability of cadaver kidneys: a function of public and physician education and optimal organization of organ harvesting, improved methods of preservation, matching and distribution.

Comparing the present situation of kidney transplantation in Western Europe with that in the United States and Japan, some differences can be pointed out. In fact, in the latter country cadaver grafts supply only 10-15% of the total, the rest coming from living donors. This keeps the number of transplants very low, so that in Japan only 1190 kidney transplants have been performed between 1956 and 1978 (K. Ota, Trans. ISAO, 1979). In the United States, the situation is reversed, but still about 30% of grafts come from living donors. Western Europe, on the contrary, relies mainly on cadaver kidneys and this is evident from Table 8 where the transplantation rate in european countries in 1979 is reported.

In Europe, during the late 1960's, several organisations have been set up for the management of kidney transplantation, of which the principal ones are:

- <u>Eurotransplant</u>, in which Austria, Belgium, Germany and The Netherlands participate, and which also serves other unassociated West European Countries such as Italy, Spain and Greece, and East European countries such as the Democratic Republic of Germany and Poland.

- France Transplant, which exchanges information with Swiss Transplant and Hispano Transplant.
- UK Transplant Service, serving also the Irish Republic.
- Scandiatransplant, which links Sweden, Norway, Denmark, Finland, Iceland and some centres of northwest Germany.

These organisations are, of course, cooperating together and this has helped to make kidney transplantation rather successful in Europe.

In fact, the main purpose of such organisations are, using the words of Eurotransplant:

- to maximize the survival time of transplanted organs through tissue typing and matching,
- to create a structure in which as many patients as possible who need an organ for transplantation will receive an appropriate organ as soon as possible and
- to achieve, by the creation of an efficient structure, a high utilization rate of available organs.

To achieve these aims, the organization has:

1. established a network of laboratories for donor and recipient typing and cross matching purposes,
2. standardized techniques and reagents,
3. set up a central registration of potential recipients that can be daily up-dated and supply a regular feed-back of information,

4. developed a system of selection procedures that function with the shortest delay and the least effort, and
5. created a communication center with expertise in organizational aspects of donor procurement, organ transportation, transplantation and financing.

Figure 8 gives the evolution of kidney transplantation as recorded by the four major European organizations, and the steady increase of transplants performed is evident.

Nevertheless, the number of patients waiting for a transplant also increases continuously and according to the 1979 Eurotransplant Annual Report the number of patients on the waiting list increased in 1979 by 25% over 1978, reaching a total of 2581! A similar situation is recorded by the other organizations and the waiting time is still too long.

According to Scandiatransplant, the waiting time in 1980 was 8.9 months, down from 9.4 for the previous year. On the other hand, Eurotransplant recorded on 1979 an average waiting time of 24 months, which is certainly due in fact to the very careful selection of the recipient and to the Urgency Code System, adopted by Eurotransplant for selecting the patients, and which foresees different waiting times according to the degree of urgency identified. This system certainly increases the probability of success of the transplant, and a careful selection of the recipients is to be recommended (in some countries this is not strictly followed, and this is one of the reasons for increased risk of rejection). However, in the meantime, the maximum effort should be made to reduce the waiting list, since many patients die before receiving their transplant.

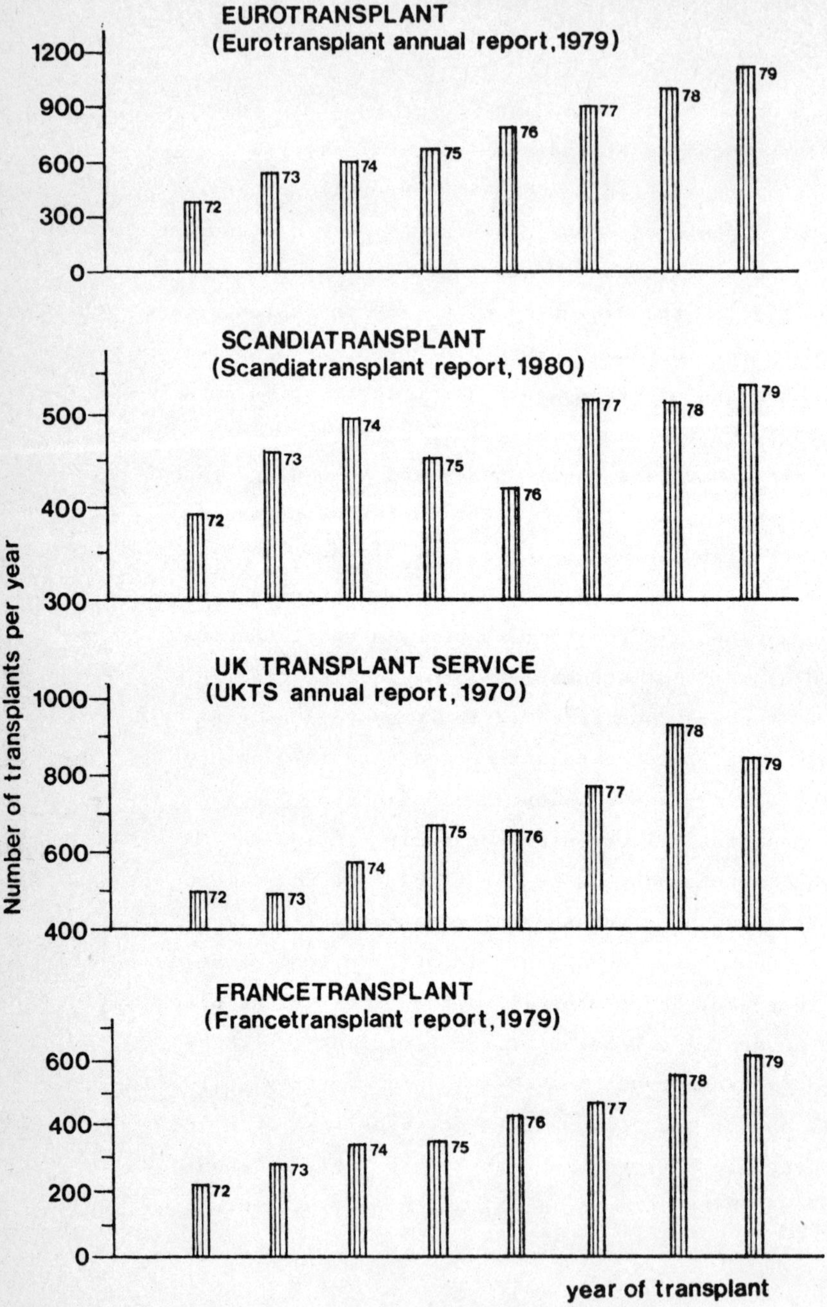

Figure 8 - Evolution of kidney transplant in Western Europe, according to the four major organizations dedicated to the management of transplantation.

In effect, in principle, the medico-surgical transplantation groups, the histocompatibility laboratories and the various organisations in the West European Countries, are well capable of handling a larger number of patients. The limiting factor for renal transplantation is the lack of cadaver kidneys.

Many factors hinder the more widespread acceptance of organ donation and people should be made aware of the benefits of transplantation in order to favour the harvesting of organs from cadavers.

The most efficient way of increasing the number of cadaver kidneys available for transplantation is to improve the relationship between the medico-surgical transplant groups and the medical and surgical departments where neurological deaths are seen. Moreover clear legislation should be prepared to regulate organ removal from cadavers. In France a law effective since April 1978 allows a surgeon to harvest organs on all cadavers except when the patient or his family has expressed written opposition. A similar law is close to be adopted in Belgium.

In other countries, such as Italy, where it is still under preparation, a similar legislation has not yet been implemented and this is one of the reasons which has hindered a wider use of kidney transplantation.

Transplants of a live donor kidney from a close blood relative give a reasonably predictable promise of functional graft survival for at least 6 to 8 years (B.T. Burton et al. Proc. 2nd Meeting ISAO, 1979). The functional survival of cadaver grafts, on the contrary, is poorer, but careful selection of the recipient can increase the probability of success. In this respect Europe is superior to the United States where the rejection rate in the case of cadaver kidneys is considerably higher, and the most recent data indicate for Europe a graft survival of about 60% at 2 years (Eurotransplant Annual Report, 1979).

Patient survival is also improved by appropriate management of kidney transplantation and in the Eurotransplant area the overall data show that the 5-year patient survival is 70% (Figure 9).

Similar results are found also in the areas covered by the other three major European organisations, which confirms the importance of a centralised organisation for the management of kidney transplantation by which medico-surgical transplantation groups are strictly linked with histocompatibility laboratories.

Recently, it has been found that blood transfusions antecedent to kidney transplantation can improve graft survival (J. Jeckel et al., Proc. EDTA, 1980), and therefore an appropriate programme of blood transfusions could increase the probability of success.

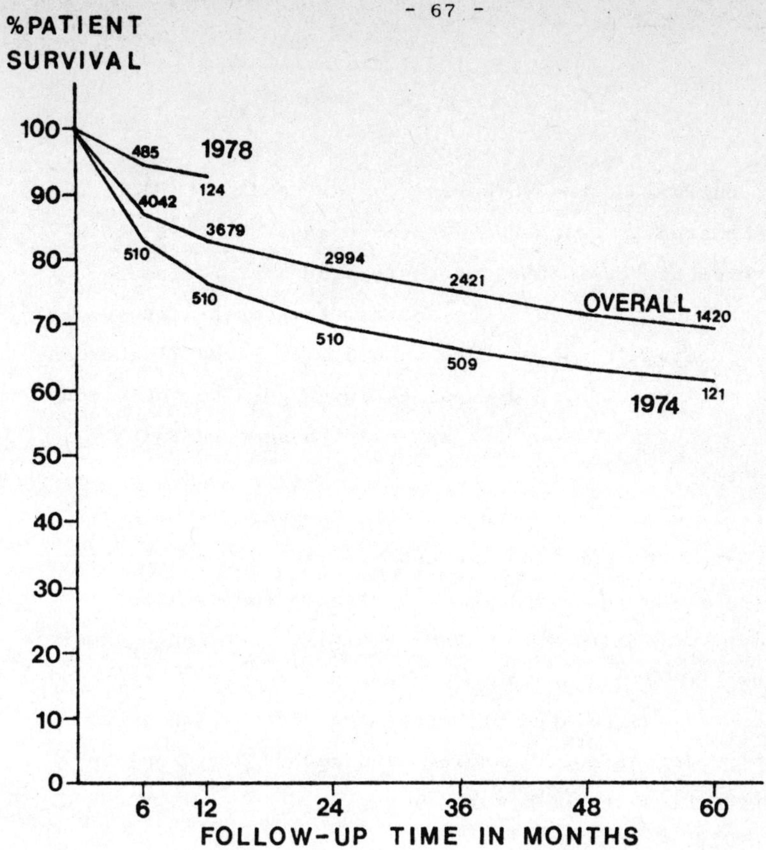

Figure 9 - Patient survival related to year of transplantation in the Eurotransplant area. (Numbers are the patients at risk).

Source : Eurotransplant Annual Report, 1979.

In conclusion, though besides organisational problems, also other aspects related to kidney transplantation, notably improvements of immunosuppressive therapy, recipient rehabilitation etc. need to be solved, this treatment modality for end stage renal disease should find steadily increasing application, even on grounds of lower cost to the community of successful kidney transplantation compared with dialytic therapy.

Therefore, the European Economic Community should encourage closer cooperation amongst the various organisations already existing in Europe, should promote the creation of similar associations in those countries where such organisations are missing, and should sponsor research programmes in fields related to kidney transplantation such as organ preservation, immunology and methodology for the early prediction of graft survival.

VIII. FUTURE DEVELOPMENT OF THERAPY FOR END-STAGE RENAL DISEASE

Dialytic therapy for the treatment of chronic renal failure is a typical example of halfway technology, since although it has made life possible for patients suffering from a fatal illness, it does not bring the patient back into a healthy status.

During the last decade remarkable improvements in the management of uremic patients and in the understanding of the pathophysiology of end-stage renal disease have occurred. Nevertheless, many side effects and weaknesses are still associated with this treatment modality and the present status of uremic therapy seems to have reached a plateau in its evolution.

The two most recent innovations in the field are haemofiltration and continuous peritoneal dialysis (CAPD and CCPD), but these too tackle only the problem of uremic wastes, which is only one aspect of uremia, and they too have their own limitations and drawbacks.

As already mentioned earlier in this report, after the enthusiasm that followed the first experiments, haemofiltration has not maintained the initial promises of providing a much more efficient therapy for the treatment of end-stage renal disease.

Haemofiltration seems to give a better regulation of blood pressure and better welfare of the patient (E. Quellhorst et al., Clin. Nephrol., 1979; S. Nakagawa, Artif. Organs, 1980), nevertheless the superiority, if any, of haemofiltration over haemodialysis is not dramatic and in consideration also of its higher cost and complexity, it is thought that, in its present form, haemofiltration will remain a relatively little used procedure for the treatment of uremia.

Continuous peritoneal dialysis seems more promising. Of the two modalities proposed, continuous ambulatory peritoneal dialysis (CAPD) and continuous cycling peritoneal dialysis (CCPD), the former, which was started first, has become fairly widely used in a relatively short time (2.4% of european patients were treated in 1980 with this technique). Patients enjoy being free from dialysis machines, feel less sick (P.C. Farrel, Amer. Soc. Artif. Intern. Organs, 1979) and the cost is relatively low. However, as already pointed out, peritonitis, which occurs approximately twice a year in each patient, and excessive weight gain, due to the daily absorption of 100 g of carbohydrate, present in the dialysate, with consequent effect on triglycerides, make the picture less rosy.

In fact, the cost due to peritonitis in terms of hospitalization has been well documented and increased triglyceridemia can enhance the incidence of cardiovascular complications. These problems, and other as well, such as those associated with necessity of introducing into the abdomen a relatively large volume of fluid, must be solved before the technique is more widely adopted. Therefore, taking into account the pressure for a reduction in the costs associated with present dialytic therapy and of the necessity to make this treatment modality available to an ever larger number of patients, in the short-medium term efforts need to be focused on the improvement of those technical and clinical aspects which would lessen, if not eliminate, some of the drawbacks associated with dialytic therapy.

Certainly helpful would be the production of more permeable membranes, thereby eliminating the controversy about middle molecules. Also better dialysers are needed, since an improved flow distribution of both blood and dialysate (with the current dialysers the surface area is not entirely used), would improve the efficiency of the dialysers and reduce their size. If a substantial reduction of the cost of dialysers cannot be achieved, safe, reusable, dialysers should be developed.

The development of less thrombogenic materials and of new methods for anticoagulant therapy should be also considered, since the problems associated with the thrombogenicity of the artificial materials and the unwanted side-effects due to the use of heparin, are detrimental to the well being of the patient and may exclude patients from dialytic treatment altogether in some cases.

Improvements should also be sought in the composition, preparation and delivery of the dialysis solution. Strict control of water quality should be introduced, and the treatment of water by reverse osmosis and by ion exchange resins should be recommended. Also the purity of the salts used for the preparation of dialysate should be taken into account, since too high a level of impurities makes a nonsense of water purification, so that a more strict control on the selection of reagents used should be enforced.

The search for efficient systems of dialysate regeneration is another field of investigation, since it would permit a reduction in the volume of dialysate required and simplify the development of portable equipments.

Particular attention should be devoted to the early identification of the pathological causes of end-stage renal disease in order to identify the subjects at risk, with a view to introducing preventive measures.

This means an effort toward education of both the public and the doctors, and the development of an optimal health care organization. However prompt diagnosis would certainly be of great help and in many cases would prevent the degeneration of illness to the point of no-return.

The development of better drugs for the control of hypertension would be welcomed not only in the treatment of cardiovascular disorders but also in the treatment of end-stage renal disease, since hypertension is considered to be one of the major causes of accelerated arteriosclerosis, the first killer amongst uremic patients.

It would be particularly helpful in some cases, to reduce the external factors which either contribute to or aggravate chronic renal failure.

Smoking, for example, has being identified as an important risk factor for uremic patients (H. Haire, Am. Soc. Artif. Intern. Organs, 1976) and it should not be impossible to keep this factor under control.

Drug nephropathy is another example in which public action could be effective. In fact, the increase in this syndrome has been associated with an indiscriminate use of drugs (generally analgesics), particularly apparent in some countries, and a campaign against drug abuse and more strict control on drug sale, would certainly reduce substantially the incidence of drug nephropathy.

Other modalities of dialytic therapy should also be sought, and in this respect it would be worthwhile to investigate the possibility of extracting the uremic wastes from blood or intestinal fluids by specific, as well as aspecific, sorbents.

Specific sorbents, such as aluminium hydroxide and sodium polystyrene sulfonate resins have already found clinical application for the gastrointestinal removal of excess phosphate and potassium ions, respectively.

Recently, it has been reported that lavage of the gastrointestinal tract after ingestion of a large volume (about 7 litres) of a solution of mannitol, has resulted in an improvement of the condition of uremic patients (T.K. Young et al., Int. J. Artif. Organs, 1979).

This procedure, although simple and not very expensive, is certainly not very pleasant for the patient, and active investigation has been devoted to the search for sorbents which, taken orally in relatively small amount, could be excreted with bound uremic wastes.

Many types of non specific sorbents for urea have been tested, from activated charcoal (J.F. Winchester, Artif. Organs, 1977) to non-digested, natural polymers, such as locust bean gum (H. Yatzidis et al., Clin. Nephrol., 1979; Dial. TRansplant., 1980) and oxidized polysaccharides such as oxystarch (C. Giordano et al., Artif. Organs, 1977) or oxycellulose (C. Giordano, Clin. Nephrol., 1979).

These attempts, and many others, have been thoroughly reviewed recently (C. Giordano, Sorbents and Their Clinical Applications, 1980). However, besides some disconfort for the patient, such as the problems associated with the ingestion of such substances and intestinal disturbances, even the most active systems, such as oxystarch, do not remove more than 15 grams of urea per 200-250 grams of binder, which is not sufficient for intestinal use.

Some of these sorbent systems could be used for the development of devices for dialysate regeneration, but effective urea removal must be regarded as a largely unresolved problem and the search for more efficient sorbent systems should continue.

A particularly attractive approach has been proposed lately, which could provide continuous purification from uremic wastes.

The rationale of this approach is based on the observation that many rumen bacteria and soil bacteria are grown with ammonia of urea (K. Setala et al., Proc. EDTA, 1972). Ruminants recycle nitrogenous wastes with the assistance of nitrogenous bacteria. Therefore, specific strains of microorganism could be used either internally or extracorporeally (biological reactors) for the removal of uremic wastes.

It has already been proved that oral doses of soil bacteria have resulted in a decrease in blood urea nitrogen and serum creatinine level of uremic patients (K. Setala, Kidney Int., 1978).

So far there is too little information about this approach, but its potentialities are intriguing.

In fact, besides a search for more appropriate microorganisms, or mixtures of them, more specific microorganisms might be produced taking advantage of the possibilities offered by genetic engineering. This might make possible the manipulation of non-pathogenic microorganisms to transform them into species more efficient in recycling nitrogenous wastes, as well as able to synthesize aminoacids from guanidines, phenols and creatinine.

Unfortunately, whatever success will be achieved with the approaches outlined above, only the excretory function of kidney will be subserved, and the problem of the treatment of end-stage renal disease will be only lessened.

Moreover, no dramatic breakthrough can be expected in the near future in the field of kidney transplantation.

Therefore, while waiting for the problems related to kidney transplantation, such as organ harvesting and preservation, rejection etc., which are common also to any other organ transplants, to be solved, methods for developing true artificial organs should be explored. This approach is likely to become more viable during the next two decades.

The development of an artificial kidney is certainly not easy, and in many respects is more difficult than developing an artificial heart, since normal kidneys perform, continuously, a complex series of functions including:

- control of water balance
- control of electrolytes
- control of acid-base balance
- removal of wastes
- production and degradation of hormones
- participation in protein anabolism and catabolism.

An artificial kidney should, therefore, simulate the sophistication of kidneys and mimic also their endocrine and protein metabolism functions.

The development of such an artificial kidney might be achieved in two steps.

The first, would be the development of a wearable, semi-bionic kidney, which uses cybernetic regulation, with a blood sensor that regulates the infusion of electrolytes, hormones, proteins, amino acids, and vitamins as needed, in combination with a dialysis filter to eliminate waste.

The second would be an implantable bionic kidney. The problem has been discussed at the ASAIO Meeting in 1979 (Panel Conference: Hybrid Artificial Organs), where it was suggested that a bionic kidney could be made by implanting a dialyser in the abdomen of a patient, seeded with renal tubular cells. Such a dialyser should be able to remove toxins, while the growing cells would reuse and catabolize or anabolize hormones and proteins. Combining this system with an exchangeable sorbent cartridge to accumulate waste, it should be possible to improve greatly the life and longevity of a patient who has lost his kidney.

IX. THERAPEUTIC HAEMAPHERESIS

The concept of removing toxic substances from the blood as a therapeutic treatment is certainly not new and dialysis is at present the most widely used procedure of blood detoxification.

However, the principle of dialysis itself dictates the shortcoming of this treatment method, since only molecules of limited molecular weight can be removed.

The success obtained by dialysis in improving the condition of uremic patients proves that this technique works. However, with the introduction of the "middle molecules" theory, its inability to remove all toxic substances contributing to the uremic syndrome, has been suggested.

As a consequence, membranes of higher porosity and efficiency have been sought. Neverthless, dialysis will always fall short of complete success in cases where toxic substances fail to pass through the membrane, either because of their very high molecular weight or because they are bound to plasma proteins.

To overcome these problems, the direct treatment of whole blood has been considered, but though haemoperfusion over activated charcoal has proved to be succesful in treating some types of drug intoxication, the wider use of this technique has been hampered because of potentially life-threatening thrombocytopaenia and embolization due to charcoal particles release.

With the advent of procedures to enhance biocompatibility and reduce the danger of embolization, haemoperfusion has been used with success in the treatment of certain types of poisoning (J.F. Winchester et al., Artif. Organs, 1978; E. Piskin et al. Intern. J. Artif. Organs, 1981).

However, the possibility of particle release remains a problem, and traumatic effects to blood cellular components during haemoperfusion can also occur.

Moreover, charcoal is an insufficiently specific sorbent, so that in the constant search for more efficient systems of blood detoxification, a novel procedure of blood letting has given rise to new hopes.

This has been made possible by the advent of automated cell separators, at first used in blood centres for the collection of granulocytes and platelets from normal donors.

However, their availability in general hospitals has led to therapeutic use of this technique which, depending on the blood component considered, is currently known as:

- Cytopheresis (separation of cellular components of blood)
- Plasmapheresis (substitution or treatment of plasma).

Cytopheresis was the first therapeutic application of cellular separators (M. Benbunam et al. Nouv. Rev. Franc. Haemat., 1973) and has been used in the therapy of various diseases, for example certain types of granulocytopaenia (M. Wieckowicz, Transfusion, 1976).

Plasmapheresis, intended both as plasma exchange and as plasma treatment, seems more interesting, and might have a wider application since this detoxification modality has shown promising results in the therapy of a large spectrum of diseases.

Particularly attractive are the possibilities of treating autoimmune disorders and success in this direction would be a real breakthrough since 15% to 20% of all hospital admissions are for autoimmune disorders; arthritis alone affects about 1% of the world population!

Table 9 shows most of the diseases which could be treated with haemapheresis, and considering that at the present the majority of them do not respond to conventional therapy the potentialities of plasmapheresis are enormous, so that this report will deal essentially with this procedure.

TABLE 9

Examples of diseases which could be treated by haemapheresis

Plasmapheresis	Cytopheresis
- Myasthenia gravis	- Leukemia Acute and Chronic
- Macroglobulinemia	- Lymphophoresis
- Cryoglobulinaemia	- Cutaneous T-cell Lymphoma
- Thyroid Storm	- Platelet Thrombocytosis
- Multiple Myeloma	- Sickle Cell Anaemia
- Goodpasture's Syndrome	- Polycythemia
- Systemic Lupus Erythematosus	- Paroxysmal Nocturnal Haemoglobinuria
- Rheumatoid Arthritis	
- Pemphigus Vulgaris	
- RH Disease	
- Acquired Anti-Factor VIII	
- Guillain Barré Syndrome	
- Familial Hypercholesterolemia	
- Thrombotic Thrombocytopenic Purpura	
- Idiopathic Rapidly Progressive Glomerulonephritis	
- Hyperviscosity Syndrome	
- Renal Graft Rejection	
- Drug Overdose	
- Multiple Sclerosis	

Plasma exchange was the first method of plasmapheresis to be used. It consists in removing the patient's plasma which contains the damaging agent, and replacing it with physiological fluids.

Usually the exchange volume varies between two and four litres and in this case a solution of correct electrolyte composition(Na^+, Ca^{++}, K^+, Cl^-), and adequate colloid activity (albumin), is enough for replacement.

However, when plasma exchange is performed frequently or when large volumes of plasma are exchanged, a plasma protein fraction is also added to the replacement fluid. Such an addition increases very much the cost of the treatment, and can cause unwanted side-effects, such as hepatitis.

The separation of blood is carried out by centrifugation in an extracorporeal circuit, using heparin or citrate for anticoagulation. Currently there are two types of cell separator. In one case, separation is carried out in a continuous flow system, and the main advantages of this procedure, are the small extracorporeal blood volume (about 300 ml), better patient tolerance and the large volume of blood processed in a short time.

In the other case, the separation is carried out with an intermittent flow system, in which up to one litre of blood may be held in the extracorporeal circuit. The advantages of this procedure are mainly portability and simple priming, but, on the other hand, this method may cause some disconforts associated with removal of quite a large quantity of blood, and since the volume of plasma exchanged each time is small, the treatment becomes tedious and it is sometimes poorly tolerated by the patient.

Recently, plasma exchange has been simplified by the introduction of filters for the separation of plasma from whole blood, which has made the use cell separators unnecessary (K. Ouchi et al., Trans. ASAIO, 1978). In fact, in this case the blood of the patient is circulated extracorporeally through the filter, much as in haemodialysis, and plasma is separated from cellular elements by a membrane of very high porosity (cellulose di-acetate, or polypropylene).

Also with this procedure it is necessary to replace the plasma with a biological fluid.

Interest in the possibilities offered by plasmapheresis is clearly indicated by the exponential growth of publications on this subject during the last few years.

A survey of the literature on therapeutic plasmapheresis has shown that more than 80% of the most important publications (560) on this subject were published between 1978 and 1980, with 1980 accounting for about 40% of the total (H.J. Gurland et al., in Therapeutic Plasma Exchange 1981).

Most of the results reported have been obtained using the cell separator but in the last two years the use of plasma filters became more common.

Since it was first started, therapeutic plasmapheresis, usually associated with chemotherapy, such as immunosuppressive therapy in the treatment of autoimmune disorders, has proved to be of help in the treatment of many diseases which are resistant to conventional therapy.

Beneficial effects from plasmapheresis have been claimed in the treatment of circulatory diseases such as Goodpasture's syndrome (H.O. Senekjian et al., Arch. Intern. Med. 1980; W.A. Briggs et al. Medicine 1979), Raynaud's disease (G. Talpos et al. Lancet, 1978) or polyartheritis nodosa (J.M. Chaloping et al., Brit. Med. J., 1980), and thrombotic thrombocytopenic purpora (A. Shinoda et al., Artif. Organs, 1981).

Neurological disorders, such as myasthenia gravis, have also been successfully treated by plasma exchange (J. Newson-Davis et al., Neurology, 1978) and plasmapheresis has been experimented also in the treatment of multiple sclerosis (P.C. Dare et al., Neurology, 1980; H.L. Weiner et al., ibid., 1980). Diseases associated with circulating immune complexes, such as lupus erithematosus (J.V. Jones et al., Lancet I, 1976) or multiple myeloma (P.K. Ray et al., Cancer, 1980) have also been treated by plasmapheresis with encouraging results.

However, it should be emphasized that all these studies remain experimental and the benefits claimed in initial optimistic reports may not withstand the test of time.

Various critical surveys of the literature published on therapeutic plasmapheresis have been already carried out to assess the efficacy of this treatment modality (J.P. Ibister, Med. J. Austr., 1979; P.C. Raich et al., Wis. Med. J., 1979). The results of the survey presented by Prof. Gurland at the last ASAIO meeting (H.J. Gurland et al., Proc. ASAIO, 1981) were particularly interesting.

In his review, Gurland has classified the diseases treated by plasma exchange according to their clinical outcome, as reported in the literature.

We have summarized the results in Table 10 (the diseases have been reported also according to the International Classification of Diseases (8th Rev.) to help their identification) and, as can be seen, the effectiveness of plasmapheresis in treating quite very serious and life threatening diseases, has been established.

Nevertheless, the outcome remains unpredictable, since many patients recover and others do not. Also the effect of supplementary medicaments given during treatment has not been fully established. In the same way the effect of the frequency and duration of the treatment itself is not yet fully defined.

Therefore, an aggressive effort to assess the real value and the limitations of plasmapheresis, hopefully aided by the introduction of a protocol for the management of this treatment modality (including chemotherapy, duration etc.) should be promoted. This would facilitate a comparison of the results obtained by different scientists, as well as investigations leading to a better understanding of the pathophysiology of the various disorders. It might lead ultimately to the development of a simpler and less expensive procedure for treatment.

TABLE 10

Classification of diseases treated by plasmaexchange*

Class-ification	Disease Treated	International Classification of Diseases (8th Rev) Code No	Section
Proven	Goodpasture's Syndrome	446.1	VII "Diseases of the circulatory system"
	Myasthenia Gravis (includes myasthenic crisis)	733	XIII "Diseases of the musculoskeleta system and connective time"
	Hyperparathyroidism (includes thyroid storm)	252	III "Endocrine, nutritional and metabolic disease"
	Exogenous Intoxication	E850-E877	E XVII "Accidents, poisonings and violence (external causes)
Justified	Haemophilia (includes haemophilia with antibody to factor VIII)	286	IV "Diseases of blood and blood-forming organs"
	Paraproteinemia	275.9	III "Endocrine, nutritional and metabolic diseases"
	Thrombotic Thrombocytopenic Purpura	446.4	VII "Disease of the circulatory system"
	Acute nephritis (includes immune-complex rapid progressive glomerulonephritis)	580	X "Diseases of genito-urinary system"
	Pemphigus Vulgaris	694	XII "Diseases of the skin and subcutaneous tissue"
Promising	Guillain Barre Syndrome	354	VI "Diseases of the nervous system and sense organs"
	Rheumatoid Arthritis	712.3	XIII "Diseases of the musculo-skeletal system and connective tissue"
	Systemic Lupus Erythematosus	734.1	XIII " " "
	Rhesus Disease	775	XV "Certain causes of perinatal morbidity and mortality"
Possible	Hypercholesterolemia (includes familial)	272	III "Endocrine, nutritional and metabolic diseases"
	Complications of Trans-planted Organs (includes renal allograft rejection		XVII "Accidents, poisonings and violence (Nature of injury)"

*Source: H J Curland (Trans. Asaio, 1981)

In fact, in many of attempts so far carried out, plasmapheresis has been administered without a complete understanding of the pathophysiology of the disease treated. The exchange of plasma has sometimes been a rather crude, little justified procedure.

Only when there is a demonstrable circulating factor which is directly responsible for a certain illness, is plasma exchange a logical and often effective therapy.

The introduction of a filter for plasma separation has already simplified the management of plasmapheresis, but the replacement of plasma with biological fluids is still necessary. Therefore the treatment is sometimes plagued by the complications associated with fluid replacement such as hepatitis, or changes in haematologic and biomedical parameters of varying intensity (M. Chopek et al., Transfusion, 1979).

Moreover, plasma exchange is a very expensive therapy (more than 1000 US dollars per session), and before it can be widely used its costs must be reduced, particularly because its value is still ill defined.

Selective removal of target plasma components, either through on-line or off-line systems, would permit use of the patient's own plasma, and would at the same time be less expensive and more efficient than conventional plasma exchange.

The introduction of membranes for plasma separation has shown the way to achieve these goals.

In fact, currently available systems allow the on line treatment of up to seventeen litres of plasma per session (Y. Asanuma et al., Trans. ASAIO, 1980). The removal from blood of toxic substances could be carried out by using first an on-line plasma filter to separate plasma from cellular elements, and then a system of "reactors" and membranes, or a series of membranes of different porosity, for the selective removal of plasma factors.

In this way it should be possible to treat abnormalities associated with albumin-bound toxins or immunological disorders (P.S. Malchesky et al., Haemoperfusion 1980; Y. Asanuma et al., Proc. ESAO, 1979).

In fact, a two membrane system has been already used, with clinically favourable results, in the treatment of various autoimmune diseases, hyperviscosity syndrome and extensive carcinoma (T. Agishi et al., in Plasma Exchange, 1980). Again, by using a plasma filter and a cryogel filter, severe rheumathoid arthritis has been successfully treated (P.S. Malchesky et al., Artif. Organs, 1980).

In the latter case, the plasma filter had a porosity of about 0.4 μ, while the cryofilter had a porosity of 0.1 - 0.2 μ so that immune complexes and gamma globulin fractions were eliminated, while albumin and other low-molecular weight plasma components were returned to the patient.

This system has been developed into a commercial machine (Cryomax), presented by Parker Biomedical (USA) at the beginning of 1981.

An evolution of the above approach leads one to the so-called "cascade membrane system", in which membranes of various porosity are used in sequence to remove macromolecules, with molecular weights ranging from few million daltons to under 100.000 daltons, selectively from plasma.

In Table 11 a breakdown of the porosity requirements for "cascade membranes" is given. Modern technology should be able to meet these.

TABLE 11

Porosity requirements of membranes for selective removal of macromolecules by plasmafiltration

Membrane Porosity (μ)	Approximate Molecular Weight of Macromolecules Still in the Plasma (Daltons)
0.2 - 0.6	$>$1,000,000 (Immune Complexes)
0.06 - 0.2	100,000-1,000,000 (Globulins)
0.01 - 0.06	$<$100,000 (Albumin)

Besides the "cascade membrane" approach, which, given the correct set of membranes, is probably the simplest one for blood detoxification, other ways have been sought to eliminate specific plasma components.

A very popular approach has been the development of "reactors", in which the toxic substances are eliminated either by simply trapping them as with charcoal, but more selectively, or through a reaction, usually enzymatic, by means of which the circulating humoral factor is transformed into a harmless product.

The search for reactors capable of removing immune complexes has been particularly active since in current immunology it is widely accepted that these macromolecules play a central phlogistical role in many phenomena associated with inflammatory processes. Processes associated for example, with systemic lupus erithematosus and poststreptococcal glomerulonephritis, and with certain malignant diseases.

The mechanism is not clear, but it is thought the tissue injury is due to immune complex deposition via immunoglobulin or complement receptors (W.P. Reed et al., Adv. Int. Med., 1977; S.R. Hollàn et al.,; Haematologia, 1978/79, H.H. Sedlacek et al., Klin. Wochensch.; 1980, J.F. Bach, Rev. Praticien, 1980).

A survey of the most recent literature has shown that various sorbent systems have been developed for the selective removal of toxins from plasma, and in Table 12 the most interesting approaches are reported, some of which have already been tested on a few patients with favourable results.

A particularly interesting specific adsorbent was presented at the last ASAIO meeting (G. Schmer et al., Abstract ASAIO, 1981).

TABLE 12

Selection of the most interesting sorbent systems for selective removal of humoral factors, and diseases likely to be treated

SORBENT	FACTOR REMOVED	PRIMARY DISEASE AND/OR INTERMEDIATE DISORDER TREATED	REFERENCE
USP-Charcoal, coated glass beads	Bile acids	Primary biliary cirrhosis Arteriohepatic dysplasia (Alagille's syndrome)	Lauterburg (1980)
Dowex and XAD resins	Bile acids Acute drug overdose	Liver disease Coma by drug intoxification	Weston (1975) Rosenbaum (1979)
Heparin-agarose	Lipoproteins	Homozygous familial hypercholesterolemia	Lupien (1980) Burgstaler (1980)
Specific anti-bodies covalently bound to Sepharose	Antiphenobarbital antibodies	Drug intoxification (speculative)	Callegaro (1981)
DNA Collodion Charcoal	Antibody to single stranded DNA and immune complexes	Systemic lupus erythematosus	Terman (1979)
Staphylococcus Aupous Protein A immobilized on acrylic beads or Sephadex	IgG immunoglobulins	Human multiple myoloma " colonic carcinoma " autoimmune haemolytic anemia " anti-acetylcholine receptor antibody	Ray (1980) Bansal (1978) Pineda (1980)
		Canine mammary carcinoma " fibrosarcoma " aquamous cell carcinoma " haemangiopericytoma	Terman (1981)
Human A and B antigen covalently bound to crystaline silica	Anti-A anti-B isoglutinins	Human bone marrow trans-plantation between ABO blood-group incompatibility	Bensinger (1981)

This system depends on red cell ghosts, treated with glutaraldehyde, which can selectively adsorb complement factors. This sorbent has been tested with sheep, by extracorporeal blood circulation through a plasma filter, and the complement level was found to have been lowered by an average 40% in 2 hours. Since numerous diseases like rheumatoid arthritis, immunovasculitis and lupus nephritis, are mediated by the complement system, the possibilities of this sorbent should be thoroughly investigated.

As already pointed out, selective removal from plasma of circulating factors directly responsible of certain illness, could also be acheived by "bio-reactors" incorporating immobilized enzymes (H. Hyden, Biomat. Med. Dev. Artif. Organs, 1980).

In effect, intravenous injections of an enzyme, for the treatment of certain diseases, is not new.

For example, the administration of asparaginase in the therapy of acute lymphatic leukaemia is known by more than a decade (Y. Ravindranath, Int. Ped. Oncol. Conf., 1981), and injections of phenylalanine ammonia-lyase have been used with interesting results in the treatment of phenylketonuria (C.W. Abell et al., Cancer Res., 1973; R.R. Fritz et al., J. Biol. Chem., 1976). However, the direct injection of an enzyme has several drawbacks, one of which is that repeated exposure to the same enzyme in this way can cause the patient to become sensitized and subject to anaphilactic shock, which is sometimes fatal.

The development of "bio-reactors", in which the enzyme is immobilized in a way that allows the enzyme to perform its action without being released into the blood stream, could overcome the problem.

Gel-immobilized microsomal enzymes have been proposed for the treatment of acute liver failure (E. Denti et al., Trans. ASAIO, 1976), and more recently, the use of an extra-corporeal reactor with immobilized L-asparaginase for the treatment of certain types of leukaemia has been reported (J.A. Jackson et al., J. Pharm. Exp. Ther. 1980).

Lately the immobilization of arginase on the inner surface of cellulose hollow fibers has been reported (V. Rossi et al., Int. J. Artif. Organs, 1981).

This result is of particular interest since it has been found that this enzyme plays a fundamental role in hyper-argininaemia, an arginase-deficiency disease, characterized by mental retardation, spastic paralysis and tremor (S.D. Cederbaum et al., Pediat. Res., 1979; K. Adriaenssens et al., Clin. Chem., 1976).

Moreover, in vitro, arginase can inhibit the growth of some malignant cells (G.A. Currie et al., Br. J. Cancer, 1978a) and therefore this system could also be used in the treatment of tumours.

Ligandin, an enzyme possessing binding properties for a large number of lipophilic compounds, including bilirubin, has also been immobilized on the inner surface of cellulose hollow fibers and this "reactor" could be helpful in the treatment of liver diseases (L. Callegaro et al., Int. Symp., 1980).

Besides those mentioned above, other methods of enzyme immobilization are known which could also be used for therapeutic purposes (T.M.S. Chang, BIomedical Application of Immobilized Enzymes and Proteins, 1977).

Amongst these, two approches seem particularly interesting for clinical applications.

In one, worked-out by Chang, the enzyme has been immobilized inside semipermeable polymer membranes of varying porosities and the possible therapeutic applications of different types of immobilized enzymes and proteins have been investigated. These results have been reviewed elsewhere (T.M.S. Chang, Biomedical Application of Immobilized Enzymes, 1977; T.M.S. Chang, Artif. Organs, 1980), and we will give here only a few examples of applications of this system.

The results of recent studies, which have demonstrated the feasibility of using artificial cells containing tyrosinase for the in vivo conversion of tyrosine and phenols in rats suffering from fulminant hepatic failure, have been very interesting (C.D. Shu et al., Int. J. Artif. Organs, 1981).

Artificial cells have also been used for the immobilization of asparaginase, and this system has been effective in the experimental suppression of lymphosarcoma (T.M.S. Chang, Nature, 1971).

Multienzyme systems have also been immobilized inside artificial cells, and in the most recently developed system, urease, glutamate dehydrogenase and transaminase have been immobilized together for the enzymatic conversion of urea (T.M.S. Chang, Proc. ISAO, 1979).

In the other approach considered, the enzyme is immobilized inside red cell ghosts (RCG) (M.M. Billah et al., Biochim. Biophys. ACTA, 1977) and Dr. Schmer, of Univ. of Washington, Seattle, has been one of the most active in using this system of immobilization.

A potent enzyme reactor has been prepared by binding urease-filled RCG to a matrix of Sephadex G-25 containing covalently bound Concovallin A, and this system has shown high efficiency for breakdown of urea to CO_2 and NH_3 (G. Schemer et al., Trans. ASAIO, 1977).

Red cell ghosts have been used also for the immobilization of asparaginase, and reactors based on this system have been successfully used in vivo, to reduce the asparagine level in sheep, obtaining a 50% decrease of this amino acid after two hours of treatment by extracorporeal circulation.

In conclusion, although so far these "reactors" have not attained regular clinical use (many problems still need to be solved, let only mention, for example, the complications associated with the sterilization of reactors containing an immobilized enzyme) the examples reported above suggest that their use for the removal from plasma of humoral factors responsible of certain diseases, could become as important therapeutic tool in the near future, especially in combination with the methods of plasma separation recently developed (H.G. Sieberth, Int. Symp., 1981).

The identification of the circulating substances responsible for specific diseases will be very important in the development of appropriate reactors.

In the case of immune complex diseases the action promoted by the World Health Organization in defining the analytical techniques which must be used to detect immune complexes in the serum of patients will be also very helpful (WHO, Technical Report Series, 1977).

At this point, however, we cannot conclude our short survey on therapeutic plasmapheresis, both as plasma exchange and plasma treatment, without a warning against its indiscriminate use.

In fact, this treatment modality could be a real breakthrough and its real value must be assessed.

As mentioned above, plasmapheresis is usually used in those cases in which conventional therapy is ineffective, but the alarming notion that this therapeutic modality is, in any case, likely to do no harm, is unacceptable and dangerous.

In fact, major complications, including death have been reported (R. Schlansky et al., Arthritis Rheum., 1981), and therefore, injudicious use of this therapy must be avoided.

Additional information about nearly all aspects of plasmapheresis and immunosuppressive agents is needed before a rational perspective can be developed regarding the role of plasmapheresis in clinical medicine.

Careful clinical trials with stringent control conditions are the most urgent requirement.

A comprehensive approach is made more difficult by the multitude of different clinical subjects, plasmapheresis schedules, choice of immunosoppressive regimes and measures of the outcome.

Hopefully, the development of new technical devices will render such research significantly less expensive by allowing selective removal of plasma components, thereby eliminating the need for the costly replacement solutions which are currently required.

However, this latter problem could be lessened if some of the complications associated with new techniques of cell culture and/or molecular biology lately developed, are solved.

In fact, the cost of the replacement solutions depends largely on their content of albumin, which must respond to very high standards of purity.

The synthesis of albumin, starting from hepatoma cell lines or from polysomes isolated from liver cells "activated" by albumin messanger RNA, has been reported (U.I. Richardson et al., J. Cell Biol., 1969; C. Sepirer et al.,

Differentiation, 1975; J.A. Peterson, Proc. Nat. Acad. Sci. USA, 1976; R.C. Garland et al., Mol. Cellular Biochem., 1981; R.E. Baker et al., J. Cell Biol., 1981). Therefore, the production of synthetic albumin could overcome the problems associated with its collection and purification so reducing the limitations which now hinder the therapeutic administration of albumin in this, and in other cases as well.

However, many and very complex problems must be solved before synthesised albumin could be used for therapeutic applications.

These include, for example, the toxicity of the starting material now employed, the reproducibility of the albumin produced, the isolation of it from the medium of reaction, and an aggressive research in this field is highly recommended.

X. COMPLICATIONS DUE TO BLOOD INTERACTION WITH ARTIFICIAL MATERIALS

The possible danger associated with the release of plasticizers from PVC tubing during haemodialysis has already been mentioned, as well as the hazard due to the presence of various impurities in the dialysate, so that it is particularly important that all materials coming in contact with blood are of the correct quality.

However, while the release of harmful substances can be reduced, if not eliminated completely, other complications are brought about simply by the exposure of blood to artificial surfaces, either extracorporeally or inside the body itself.

In fact, immediately following the contact of most artificial materials with blood, various blood components begin to adsorb to the surfaces. The interaction of plasma proteins with artificial surfaces can initiate blood coagulation, and activate the fibrinolytic systems (L. Vroman et al., Fed. Proc., 1971; S. Schiffan et al., J. Clin. Invest., 1975; J.H. Griffin et al., Proc. Natl. Acad. Sci. USA, 1976). Eventually, thrombin may be formed and adhere to the artificial surfaces in an active form (S.F. Mohammad et al., Proc. Natl. Acad. Sci. USA, 1976).

Following protein adsorption, blood cells are also adsorbed on the protein layer. In addition leukocytes and platelets frequently adhere in large numbers (R.G. Mason et al., Biomater. Med. Devices Artif. Organs, 1977; S.F. Mohammad et al., Haemostasis, 1974).

Many adverse reactions follow the series of events outlined above, the most dramatic being the activation of blood coagulation and thrombus formation. Complement activation is another complication associated with the interaction of blood with artificial surfaces and complement activation by the cellulose membrane has been held responsible of leukopenia and hypoxia on patients on dialysis (A.I. Jacob et al., Kidney Trans., 1980).

Thrombus formation in patients undergoing haemodialysis is averted by using anticoagulant therapy. Heparin is the most commonly used anticoagulant today, but its use poses various problems due to bleeding, difficult dosage, and unwanted side-effects, such as reversible thrombocytopenia. Therefore, the availability of materials which could be used without heparin would be worthwhile.

The problem of enhanced thrombus formation occurs not only with haemodialysis, but also when blood comes into contact with other artificial organs and devices such as catheters, vascular shunts, artificial heart valves, artificial blood vessels, blood oxygenators, etc., so that the search for better materials is particularly active.

The first approach in the development of haemocompatible materials has been the modification of commercially available polymers.

Binding heparin to polymer surfaces has been one of the most used methods, and favourable results have obtained with this approach (V.L. Gott, Adv. Exp. Med. Biol., 1974; G. Schmer, Trans. ASAIO, 1972; R.D. Falb et al., Adv. Exp. Med. Biol., 1974; R. Larsson et al., Thrombos. Res., 1979).

Besides heparin, other substances have been used to improve the blood compatibility of commercial materials. For example urokinase (A. Sugitachi et al., Int. J. Artif. Organs, 1978), a plasminogen activator. Ditazole (W. Marconi et al., Trans. ASAIO, 1979) an antiaggregating agent, and prostaglandin (J.C. Mc Rea, et al., Trans. ASAIO, 1978; S.W. Kim et al., Proc. ISAO, 1981) have all given promising results.

New types of polymer (polyurethanes, polyion, methacrilate-types, and heparin-like polymers) have also been developed, which show interesting characteristics of blood compatibility (E. Nylas et al., J. Biomed. Mat. Res. Symp. 1977; D.J.Lyman, Pure Appl. Chem., 1978; M. Sorm et al., J. Polym. Sci. Polym. Symp. 1979; K. Kotoaka et al., Makromol. Chem., 1980; M. Josefowicz et al., Proc. 27th Int. Symp. Macromol., 1981). However, so far, of these new materials only certain types of polyurethane (Avcothane, Biomer) have been developed beyond the experimental stage and tested in practical applications.

Amongst the commercially available materials for biomedical application, expanded polytetrafluoroethylene (PTFE) has shown reasonably good blood compatibility (S.K. Gupta et al., Am. J. Surg. 1980) and has been used successfully for vascular access (arterio-venous fistula) in haemodialysis.

However, the efforts to produce polymer or metal surfaces that in themselves are highly compatible with blood and so permit their use in artificial organs, including haemodialysers, without the addition of anticoagulant or antithrombotic agents, have met so far with failure for the most part.

The problem of blood compatibility is far from being solved, as was stressed at the last ASAIO Meeting (Anaheim, 6-8 May, 1981), where a panel conference with the title: "Blood/Material interaction, 20 years of frustration", was held. This failure is largely due to the lack of knowledge of the mechanism by which artificial surfaces activate clotting and permit adhesion and alteration of platelets and leukocytes. Increased efforts to answer this problem should be favoured.

In practice the poor blood compatibility of artificial materials, although a serious problem, can be managed by anticoagulant therapy in haemodialysis and in other situations which do not require too prolonged a contact of blood with the artificial surfaces. However this problem is much more serious if one wants to develop artificial organs for long-term implantation in the body.

Therefore, the development of biocompatible, less thrombogenic, materials should be the object of intensive research activity. A multidisciplinary approach, involving polymer chemists, chemical engineers, specialists on the physico-chemical properties of surfaces, haematologists etc., will be needed to give a high probability of success.

XI. THE STRUCTURE OF THE EUROPEAN MARKET IN THE FIELD OF BLOOD DETOXIFICATION

Currently, the market of the equipment used for blood detoxification can be identified with that of the equipment for dialysis, and in particular haemodialysis.

However, during the last two or three years therapeutic plasmapheresis has enjoyed an increasing popularity and the market of equipment for plasmapheresis seems bound to grow to a quite large size, and it is worth some attention.

Equipment for Haemodialysis

As has already been mentioned at the beginning of this report, the market for products associated with maintenance dialysis has reached a considerable size, which in Europe is estimated at around 400 million U.S. dollars for 1981.

This market, which has grown at a very high rate in the past (almost 20% a year), is now growing at a 12% to 14% annual rate. This growth will continue in the near future slowing down to about 5% toward the end of this decade.

The market is particularly lucrative, and European, American and now, Japanese companies are competing very hard to gain a substantial share of it.

Innovations are continually being introduced to keep pace with steady scientific and technological progress, and according to a survey made by the Stanford Research Institute at the end of 1979 on the structure of the U.S. medical supplies, equipment and device industries, the product life cycle in renal dialysis is around four years.

Therefore, a company which wants to remain competitive must be very flexible, and invest heavily in research, staying in close contact with physicians and other scientists involved in the field.

Until the late 1960's, American companies, with Baxter Travenol in the lead, have dominated the european market of dialysis equipment.

However, during the past decade, the european industry has gained more and more ground and now european companies have the leading position.

The equipment for dialysis consists essentially of three types of product: dialysers, dialysis monitoring equipment and blood lines.

To complete the set of products one should include also equipment for the treatment of water, medicaments, needles, etc., but the largest share of the market is covered essentially by the first three type of product, with the dialysers accounting for over 60% of the sales.

Dialysers

Currently, more than 55,000 patients are treated in Europe by haemodialysis and since almost 90% of them are treated three times a week, it is assumed that around 7,000,000 dialysers will be sold in Europe in 1981.

In consideration of the number of units sold, West Germany, France and Italy are the largest national markets with approximately 30%, 22% and 20%, respectively, of the total sales.

In a peculiar position is the United Kingdom which, in spite of the number of patients on treatment, accounts for a mere 3% of the total sales of dialysers in Europe. This is due to the policy followed by the Department of Health and Social Security, which continues to supply the dialysis centres essentially with the reusable, old, Kiil, dialysers. Price is a particularly critical factor in the UK, and re-use rates are surprisingly high in an effort to lower the costs.

In the remaining european countries, which constitute about 25% of the market, the re-use rate is usually very low and their respective share of sales is a direct function of the number of patients on treatment.

Although a quite large number of companies are competing in the european market, currently almost 80% of sales are in the hands of five companies: Gambro (Sweden), Hospal (France), Travenol (USA), Bellco (Italy) and Extracorporeal (USA).

The remaining 20-25% is divided amongst Fresenius (West Germany), Organon Teknica (The Netherlands), Sorin (Italy), Braun (West Germany), Cobe (USA), Cordis (USA), Dylade (UK), and Salvia (West Germany).

Usually, in those countries where there is a strong domestic company, the market is dominated by that company, as happens in Sweden with Gambro, in France with Hospal and in Italy with Bellco. In West Germany, where Gambro (Sweden) leads the field, closely followed by Travenol (USA), the German companies, Fresenius and Braun are gaining some ground.

Table 13 represents the market distribution for dialysers in Europe as a whole, and in the three largest national markets in 1979.

TABLE 13

Distribution of the european market for dialysers by major company and by country, in 1979.

Company	Country of Origin	West Germany	France	Italy	Others (+)	Total
Gambro	Sweden	35%	18%	10%	18%	22%
Travenol	USA	29%	13%	neg.	2%	20%
Hospal(++)	France	11%	47%	34%	12%	22%
Bellco	Italy	2%	8%	45%	5%	13%
Extracorporeal	USA	2%	8%	6%	6%	5%
Other	-	21%	6%	5%	30%	18%

(+) Includes United Kingdom, Austria, Scandinavia, Benelux, Ireland, Switzerland, Portugal, Spain, Greece.

(++) Includes also Hospal Dasco.

As can be seen, the first three companies are dominating the field, with similar shares of the total, but generally they have a quite different weight in the various countries.

Hospal owes its position essentially to sales in France and Italy (in Italy it also operates a joint venture with Dasco the italian subsidiary of Sandoz). Gambro relies heavily on the German market where almost 50% of its sales take place.

Similarly Travenol, which fared poorly in Italy, was strong in the lucrative West Germany market, and had a quite good position also in the other european countries, while Bellco relies on its strong lead in Italy.

The small United Kingdom market is not very attractive for the various companies. Dylade, lately acquired by the german Fresenius, covers approximately 60% of it and the UK based Meltec, which produces the Kiil dialysers, also has a good position.

Although some european companies sell japanese dialysers under their name, the direct presence of japanese groups is marginal. At present only Asahi and Torai have a significant share of the market.

During the last two years there have been some changes in the situation depicted in Table 13 due to the sharp decline in the sale of coil dialysers and to the increasing popularity of capillary dialysers which some companies failed to market promptly.

We do not have precise figures for 1981, but it can be said that while Gambro has kept, and even strengthned, its position, the other three major groups have lost some ground to companies such as Fresenius, Cordis, Cobe and Sorin.

A peculiar feature of the market for dialysers is that, in spite of the large number of companies producing them, currently only three materials are used for the dialysis membrane: regenerated cellulose (Cuprophan), cellulose acetate and polyacrylonitrile.

Of these, Cuprophan is by far the most used material, being employed for the preparation of almost 90% of all dialysers. Cuprophan is produced exclusively by Enka (West Germany), a member of the Akzo group (The Netherlands), but it seems that this monopoly situation does not cause any particular problems (only Asahi, in Japan, produces its own cellulose membranes, through an agreement with Enka).

Cellulose acetate is produced by Cordis Dow (USA), and it is used exclusively by this company, while polyacrylonitrile, which is the most expensive of all, is produced by Rhone-Poulenc, and used by its partner, Hospal.

Recently, C.R. Bard (USA) has developed a polycarbonate membrane but although it has been claimed that this membrane has better clearances toward middle molecules, improved blood compatibility etc., currently there are no indications of dialysers on the market using this membrane.

Dialysis monitoring equipment

The current dialysis monitoring machines are rather sophisticated pieces of equipment, which regulate the blood and dialysate flow through the dialyser. They also control venous and arterial pressure, dialysate temperature and composition, and blood leaks etc.

The newest types can use microprocessors for better operation and control and their average price is around 15,000 U.S. dollars.

The estimated life of such machines is eight years, and the market is phased on replacement of old machines and net growth in the number patients on home and hospital care.

The growth of the market for dialysis machines will certainly be affected, in one direction or the other, by future trends in continuous peritoneal dialysis and in home dialysis.

In fact, more patients on home dialysis will mean more machines, while the opposite will be true if continuous peritoneal dialysis gains favour.

However, no dramatic changes are expected for the next two or three years, and during this period the number of dialysis monitors to be sold in Europe, is expected to increase at a rate of 6-7% a year, not much different from the rate of increase experienced during the past two years (in 1981, the sale of dialysis monitor machines is estimated at around 3500-3700 units).

Like the market for dialysers, that for dialysis monitors is concentrated (some 75%) in the most populated european countries, including, this time, also the United Kingdom.

West Germany is the leading national market, accounting for 27-28% of the total, followed by France, Italy and the United Kingdom, with the 18%, 15% and 14%, respectively.

The major firms selling dialysis monitors are listed on Table 14, where it can be seen that this market is less polarized than that for dialysers, with the sales more evenly distributed amongst the various companies.

Moreover, Table 14 shows that, as is the case for dialysis, the strength of certain companies is heavily dependent on their position in a few countries. Only Gambro and Drake Willock had, generally, a constant, sizeable, presence in the majority of countries.

TABLE 14

Distribution of the European market for dialysis monitors by major company and by country, in 1979.

Company	Country of origin	West Germany	France	Italy	United Kingdom	Others (+)	Total
GAMBRO	USA	27%	14%	12%	7%	18%	18%
DRAKE WILLOCK	USA	13%	24%	10%	9%	17%	15%
COBE	USA	21%	5%	neg.	13%	9%	10%
DYALADE	U.K.	3%	4%	neg.	42%	9%	10%
TRAVENOL	USA	7%	7%	8%	11%	6%	7%
BELLCO	Italy	3%	3%	30%	neg.	5%	7%
DASCO	Italy	neg.	neg.	30%	neg.	6%	6%
NYCOTRON	Norway	6%	4%	5%	neg.	8%	5%
ABG-SEMCA	France	neg.	20%	neg.	-	3%	4%
RHONE POULENC	France	neg.	14%	neg.	neg.	2%	3%
OTHER	-	20%	5%	5%	18%	17%	15%

(+) Includes, Austria, Scandinavia, Benelux, Ireland, Switzerland, Portugal, Spain, Greece.

The current situation is not much different from that depicted on Table 14, except that Gambro, already in a leading position, is particularly aggressive and their newest machines seem to be quite successful.

Also very active are the american companies Drake Willock and Cobe and the german Fresenius, while other companies, bound to the so called "batch" machines, like Dasco, are losing ground.

Dialysis tubing

Second to dialysers in terms of money value is the market for dialysis tubing (arterial and venous lines).

In Europe, except in the U.K., disposable dialysers are normally supplied complete with blood lines, although tubing from a different manufacturer is sometimes used.

Most companies favour this trend by fixing the combined price of dialysers and lines at less than the price of these items purchased separately.

Blood lines are sold in sets, containing both arterial and venous lines, and their cost, which is different from one country to another as well as from one company to the next, ranges between 7 and 9 U.S. dollars a set.

In 1981 the european market for dialysis tubing is estimated at around 55-60 million U.S. dollars.

Table 15 shows the market distribution for blood lines in Europe on 1979 and also in this case West Germany is the leading national market with 26% of total, followed by Italy with 25%, France 22% and U.K. 7%.

The smaller size of the market in the United Kingdom is essentially due to the higher rate of re-use shown by this country also for these items.

TABLE 15

Distribution of the European market for dialysis tubing by major company and by country, in 1979.

Company	Country of origin	West Germany	France	Italy	United Kingdom	Others (+)	Total
GAMBRO	Sweden	30%	14%	9%	neg.	16%	16%
RHONE-POULENC	France	4%	40%	5%	16%	12%	14%
TRAVENOL	USA	20%	18%	neg.	neg.	15%	12%
BELLCO	Italy	3%	2%	45%	9%	10%	15%
DASCO	Italy	4%	8%	30%	9%	6%	12%
AVON	U.K.	3%	neg.	neg.	60%	25%	10%
EXTRACORPOREAL	USA	2%	2%	6%	7%	4%	4%
OTHER	-	32%	15%	5%	9%	12%	16%

(+) Includes Austria, Scandinavia, Benelux, Ireland, Switzerland, Portugal, Spain, Greece.

The figures reported in Table 15 are based on the number of sets sold, but since the prices of the sets are different from one company to another, the distribution would be somehow different if calculated on the price.

In this case Gambro would rise from 16% to 19% of the total and Bellco, which sells a larger number of lower-priced sets, would go down from 15% to 12%.

Amongst the companies listed in Table 15, Avon is the only one not selling dialysers and it owes its position essentially to the british market.

Purity, flexibility, resistance and low cost are the characteristics demanded of the material used for blood lines and polyvinylchloride is the material most commonly employed, although more expensive materials, such as silicone, are also used.

Some concern exists about the high content of plasticizer present in PVC tubing, which can be released into the blood stream. This has been blamed for the occurrence in some patients on maintenance dialysis of an illness similar to hepatitis.

The issue is still controversial but the problem exists and recently Bellco has started to market PVC lines(Pivicol) with a coextruded inner layer of polyurethane. These have been praised as being less thrombogenic and free from the possible troubles associated with plasticizer migration.

We did not consider the market for peritoneal dialysis equipment since the small number of patients treated with this procedure (around 4% of the total) makes this market very small.

It is however worth devoting a few words to continuous peritoneal dialysis because this technique could enjoy much wider use in the near future.

In fact, projections by Travenol, a leader in this field, indicate a continuous peritoneal dialysis market equivalent to 400 million U.S. dollars by 1985, while the less optimistic Abbot predicts for the same date a market of 100 millions. Probably both predictions are too optimistic since, as mentioned before, still many problems are unresolved, but certainly at the moment continuous peritoneal dialysis is getting the most attention.

In this field the market is, at present, a monopoly of american companies: Travenol and Abbot for continuous ambulatory peritoneal dialysis (CAPD) and American Medical Products Inc. for continuous cycling peritoneal dialysis (CCPD).

However the situation is moving fast and other companies are coming into the picture.In West Germany, Fresenious has started to offer a CAPD system and several large intravenous solution manufactures, some already making "regular" peritoneal dialysis solutions, are expected to enter soon. Cutter Laboratories (Bayer, West Germany), Green Cross (Japan), Pfrimmer (West Germany) and Salvia (Boeheringer Mannheim, West Germany) are possible examples.

The equipment used for CAPD is rather simple and consists in a bag for the dialysate, a catheter with an adapter, and tubing to connect the bag to the catheter. Except for the catheter, the equipment is disposable. The dialysate needs the approval of the health authorities before it may be sold.

The cost of a set is around 3 U.S. dollars, but the price can be different from one country to another. In view of the fact that the patient performs 4-5 changes a day, this procedure could become really economically important if it becomes widely used (it is estimated that, excluding the first year, when the cost is around 11.000 U.S. dollars, the annual cost of CAPD is about 5.000 U.S. dollars per patient).

Continuous cycling peritoneal dialysis (CCPD) is similar to CAPD except that it also needs a rather simple machine.

With this procedure changes of the dialytic solution are not so frequent, and therefore the danger of peritonitis, always present with any type of peritoneal dialysis, should be reduced.

This technique has been introduced very recently and we do not have precise figures of its cost, but in view of the need for a machine, it is likely to be more expensive than CAPD.

Equipment for Plasmapheresis

The market in equipment for plasmapheresis is at the moment quite small, being evaluated in Europe at around 8 million U.S. dollars.

Until very recently, the european market of cell separators was in the hands of three american companies: IBM, AMINCO (American Instruments Company) and Haemonetics.

However, during the last year an italian company,Dideco,

has introduced its own machine and in a very short time has captured most of the italian market.

The cell separators presently available are of two types, the intermittent flow centrifugation system (IFC), sold by Haemonetics, and the continuous flow centrifugation system, marketed by the other three companies.

These machines are priced around 35.000 U.S. dollars, but as with haemodialysis much of the business is in the disposable products (lines, blood bags etc.), which are sold at about 60 U.S. dollars a set.

The first application for the cell separators was in the blood banks, where these machines found their specific rôle with the introduction of new techniques for blood transfusion. Blood centres remain the primary market.

The introduction of therapeutic plasmapheresis has opened up new possibilities for these machines, which could widen their market.

However, with present-day equipment and methods, the cost of therapeutic plasmapheresis is very high (more than 1.000 U.S. dollars for each session), and it is doubtful whether this technique, in its present form, will be very widely used, at least until its value has been more firmly established.

A new, simpler, method for plasmapheresis has been introduced lately, in which blood is circulated extracorporeally through a plasma separator where the plasma is easily separated from the cellular elements of blood.

This procedure offers many advantages over the current plasma exchange modality, including a lower cost. It also seems more likely to be widely adopted because of recent trends in this field, which favour the selective elimination of toxic substances, without replacing the plasma.

Currently, there are on the market only two plasma separators, one, produced by Asahi (Japan), uses a cellulose di-acetate hollow fibre membrane, and the other, introduced very recently (Spring 1981) by Fresenius (West Germany), which use a hollow fibre propylene membrane, produced by Enka (West Germany).

The results so far obtained with this procedure have been encouraging but these filters are, at present, very expensive, (around 300-400 U.S. dollars each) and a reduction of price is certainly necessary before this technique can be widely adopted.

At the beginning of 1981, Parker Biomedical (USA) started to market a machine, Cryomax for on-line filtration with cryogelation of macromolecules (cryoglobulin etc.). This machine uses the Asahi filters and, allowing an easy control of all operations, makes plasmapheresis rather simple.

However, Cryomax is marketed at around 30.000 U.S. dollars, and this may hinder its wider use especially at the present, still experimental, stage of therapeutic plasmapheresis.

The production of membranes of various porosity and better biocompatibility will encourage the wider use of these detoxification systems, and we know that an aggressive search is being carried out, both in the industry and by academic institutions, in this direction.

Moreover, the development, also under investigation, of "reactors" to be used together with plasma separators for the removal of selected toxic substances, could widen the possibilities of plasmapheresis (intended as plasma treatment). We believe that if the preliminary results so far obtained are confirmed, plasmapheresis can become an attractive commercial proposition.

XII. CONCLUSIONS AND RECOMMENDATIONS

From our investigation it is evident that the two subjects treated have reached a rather different stage of evolution and different are the problems and perspectives associated with them.

Dialysis is now a consolidated, therapeutic practice for end-stage renal failure, requiring a multidisciplinary medical team, and which creates large demands on patients, their families, medical personnel, facilities and equipment.

On the other hand, plasmapheresis, associated with appropriate chemotherapy, is emerging as a new very promising treatment modality for a large number of diseases, but it is still at an experimental stage and its role in clinical medicine is not yet fully established.

Considering the dialytic therapy as it has emerged from our investigation, it is clear that:

1. In spite of its having being available for quite a long time, dialysis is far from being a fully refined medical treatment.

2. This technique has reached a plateau in its evolution and no substantial improvements can be forecast for the near future.
   In the meantime, no viable alternatives seem likely to emerge in the short term, so it is likely that this treatment modality will continue to be used for quite a long time.

3. Many scientists believe that transplantation and/or implantable artificial kidneys will be the ultimate solution to end-stage renal failure.
However, these are goals for the long term since many problems remain to be solved with transplantation and, moreover, there are patients who cannot have transplants at all, for example older individuals. Further, there are types of renal diseases that recurr in the transplant itself.
Implantable artificial kidneys too, are quite far away; therefore, while pursuing these goals, other problems should be tackled in the short-medium term.

4. This therapy is very expensive and while in the Western World absorbs a large share of the public budget for health care, in the rest of the world is little used, or not used at all, so that there is an increasing pressure to reduce its cost.

5. In the short-medium term, the efforts of both industry and the public institutions should be focused on reducing the costs of uremic therapy, as well as on improving those aspects of life which continue to provide medical obstacle for people living with renal shut down.
One way of reducing the costs would certainly be to reduce the number of patients. Of course, not through more restrictive selection rules (in some countries the criteria

for selecting the patients are already questionable, and a tighter policy in this respect is ethically unacceptable), but through early identification of the people at risk.

Certainly, prevention of end-stage renal disease is not easy, mostly because of the number and diversity of diseases that may lead to renal failure.

However, something can be done. The early identification and treatment of hypertension is one area where prevention might be achieved if organized screening, education and compliance are promoted successfully.

Neverthless, at present, only for a very few disorders which lead to renal failure are the aetiologic agents or events that initiate and perpetuate the disorder known. Therefore, before more logical preventive or therapeutic measures for uremia can be introduced, a good deal more research is needed in this direction.

Another possibility for an early reduction of the number of patients, could be the control of those environmental factors which lead to end-stage renal failure.

As mentioned earlier, drug nephropathy is one example, and campaigns against drug abuse and controls on drug sales, could reduce the incidence of this illness.

Minimal care dialysis units, similar to those under development in U.K. and Italy, should also be encouraged in an attempt both to reduce personnel costs and to increase the involvement of patients in their own care, which would be also beneficial.

Improvements in dialysis equipment and technology will also help both the welfare of the patients and the effort to reduce costs.
Such possibilities have been reviewed in Chapter VIII, and include the machines, the membranes and the procedure of dialysis.

6. Rehabilitation is another problem which should be considered with greater attention.
In fact, in addition to the medical complications associated with end-stage renal failure, there are other obstacles to rehabilitation:
   i. In-center schedules are often restricted to-day-time hours, which reduce patient's work opportunities.
   ii. Inadequate psychological and vocational counselling is available.
   iii. Professionals sometimes neglect to provide home dialysis training to qualified patients.
   iv. Inadequate emphasis is usually placed upon education and exercise for patients who could often be far more independent and active.
   v. Sometimes an unpalatable diet is imposed which places unrealistic restrictions on already undernourished people.

Many of these problems could easily be tackled by appropriate organization and specific programmes should be implemented in this direction.

Kidney transplantation research should also be encouraged since this is, at moment, the only way for recovering the kidney functions.

Research should be directed toward:

1. Kidney harvesting and preservation.
2. Tissue typing and matching.
3. Development of better immunosuppressive therapies.

The situation of therapeutic plasmapheresis is quite different. In fact, this treatment modality has been available since only a short time and it is still at an experimental stage.

Many hopes have been raised by the first results, but the real value of plasmapheresis as an effective therapeutic tool for the treatment of diseases not responding to conventional therapy, is still in doubt.

As already pointed out in chapter X, many problems must be solved before this therapeutic modality can become a common practice, but few points can be already highlighted:

1. Therapeutic plasmapheresis is rather expensive, especially in the form of plasma echange, when costly solutions for the replacement of plasma are necessary. Therefore, it is very likely that this latter procedure will remain relatively little used, unless safe and viable procedures for synthesizing albumin (the most expensive component of the replacement solution), will be developed. More promising seems the procedure of plasma treatment by which the toxic substances are removed selectively from plasma by extracorporeal circulation through membrane of appro-

priate porosity and/or specific, on line, "reactors".

2. The correct identification of humoral factors responsible for certain illnesses is of paramount importance, and research in this direction must be intensified, in order to develop appropriate systems for their selective removal.

3. Careful, double blind, clinical trials must be carried out to assess in which cases therapeutic plasmapheresis is really effective and in order to define a specific protocol.

4. Research for the development of simple and inexpensive equipments, appropriate materials, safe and efficient anticoagulation and immunosuppressive therapies, should be encouraged in any way.

In conclusion, it is evident that intensive research, basic as well as applied, is necessary in the field of blood detoxification and kidney transplantation, and this will require the cooperation of specialists of many disciplines.

Research in these fields is long, expensive, and in some cases of high risk, therefore the industry and public institutions, directly or through funding, must be involved in a joint effort.

In the United States, the National Institutes of Health (NIH) already sponsor most of the research programmes in biomedicine, and industries are granted tax exemptions for research in this field.

In Italy, too, the National Research Council, is sponsoring specific programmes in biomedicine, which include blood detoxification (Biomedical Technologies Dir. Prof. Donato), and similar efforts are also carried out in other european countries.

In Europe, however, the research in this field, as in many others, is too diversified, dispersed, little coordinated amongst the various countries, and it would be of great help if cooperative action could be started.

A quick survey of the current market and patent situation in the field of blood detoxification, has shown that Europe is well represented in the area of dialysis, but in plasmapheresis, which might have a sharp development in the near future, American, and now, very aggressively, Japanese companies, seem to have the lead.

However, considering the number of patents listed for each european country and those of U.S.A. and Japan, it is obvious that each european country alone cannot compete with U.S.A. and Japan.

Therefore, a joint community action is clearly needed in order to:

- mobilize competences and potentials
- coordinate activities
- support sectoral policies of the Commission.

The launching of a large scale community action needs the establishment of priorities and the careful distribution of tasks in space and time, and to be successful, it should be organized in the form of indirect action in which the research is performed by geographically scattered groups, operating under contracts.

Two fields can be identified, in which the community action would be more necessary:

i. One, could be toward organizational problems such as a better and deeper coordination amongst the european associations involved in kidney transplantation (Euro-transplants, U.K. Transplant, etc.) or disease prevention (WHO), the definition of common protocols for the management of dialysis and plasmapheresis therapies (selection of patients, standardization of the quality of dialysate composition, purity of water, schedule prescription, drug therapy, etc.), training of people.

ii. The second, would involve research more directly and in this case the community action should be aimed at basic research, in fact:

- Due to the time lag which at present occurs between the presentation of the programme and its actual starting, it is difficult to choose very applied topics. Both industrial and economic situations can be modified within this period.

- In any programme there are problems linked to patents, and these are, usually, less important for programmes dealing with basic research.
- Thirdly, most european industries are able to work on R and D programmes, but basic scientific work is often beyond their resources.

Some of the fields in which this research activity could be focused are:

- Pathogenesis of the diseases which can be treated by blood detoxification.
- The development of artificial blood(oxygen-carrier systems).
- Investigation on factors leading to successful kidney transplantation.
- Study of blood/surface interaction in order to develop more haemocompatible materials, to be used also for the production of implantable artificial organs.
- Development of bionic, artificial organs.

APPENDIX I

The following are the addresses of european research groups which appeared from our investigation to be the most active in the field.

Andreucci V.E. - Dept. Nephrology, 2nd Faculty of Medicine, University of Naples, Naples, Italy.

Bergström J. - Dept. Nephrology, St. Eriks Sjukhus, Stockholm, Sweden.

Boen S.T. - St. Lucas Hospital, Amsterdam, The Netherlands.

Bonomini V. - Dept. Nephrology and Dialysis, University of Bologna, Bologna, Italy.

Brynger H. - Dept. of Surgery I., Sahlgrenska Sjukhuset, Göteborg, Sweden.

Cameron J.S. - Renal Unit, Dept. Medicine, Guy's Hospital, London, U.K.

Cambi V. - Dept. Internal Medicine and Nephrology, University of Parma, Italy.

Crosnier J. - Dept. de Néphrologie and Laboratoire des Tissus Calcifiés Hôspital Necker-Enfants Malades, 149 rue de Sevres, 75730 Paris Cedex, 15 France.

Denti E. - Sorin Biomedica S.p.A., Saluggia, (Vercelli), Italy.

de Wardesser H.E. - Charing Cross Hospital Medical School, London, U.K.

Dzurik R. - Laboratory of Experimental Therapy, 3rd Medical Clinic,80946 Bratislava, Czechoslovakia.

Funck-Brentano J.L. - Dept. de Nephrologie and Laboratoire des Tissus Calcifiés, Hôpital Necker-Enfants Malades, 149 rue de Sèvres, 75730 Paris Cedex 15, France.

Giordano C. - Cattedra di Nefrologia Medica, First Faculty of Medicine, University of Naples, Italy.

Graf H. - 2nd Dept. of Internal Medicine University, Vienna, Austria.

Gurland H.J. - Med. Klinik I, Klinikum Grosshadern, Munich University, Munich, FRG.

Kerr D.N.S. - Dept. Medicine University of Newcastle upon Tyne, Tyne and Wear NE1 4LP, U.K.

Kokot F. - Dept. Nephrology Silesian School of Medicine, Katowice, Poland.

Legrain M. - Dialyse Informatione, Hôpital de La Pitié, Paris, France.

McGeown M.G. - Renal Unit, Belfast City Hospital, Belfast, Northern Ireland:

Madsen S. - Nephrological Department P, Rigshospitalet, Copenhagen, Denmark.

Moorhead J.F. - Dept. Nephrology and Transplantation, The Royal Free Hospital, London, U.K.

Morgensen C.E. - Second University Clinic of Internal Medicine, Dept. M., Aarhus Kommunehospital, DK-8000, Aarhus C., Denmark.

Parsons V. - King's College Hospital Renal Unit, London, SE5, U.K.

Quellhorst E.	- Nephrological Center Niedersachen, Hann, Muenden, FRG.
Remuzzi G.	- Division of Nephrology and Dialysis, Ospedali Riuniti di Bergamo, Bergamo, Italy.
Shaldon S.	- Dept. Nephrology University Hospital, Nîmes Montpellier, France.
Sieberth H.G.	- Med. Universitätsklinik,Köln, FRG.
Struyvenberg A.	- Dept. Internal Medicine, University Hospital, Utrecht, The Netherlands.
Traeger J.	- Clinique de Néphrologie et des Maladies Métaboliques, INSERM U80 Pavillon P., Lyon, France.
van Rood J.J.	- Dept. Immunohaematology and Blood Bank, University Medical Center Leiden, Leiden, The Netherlands.
Vercellone A.	- Nephrology and Dialysis Units, S. Giovanni Hospital, Medical Nephrology, University of Torino, Italy.
Wing A.J.	- St. Thomas' Hospital, London SEI 7EH, U.K.
Yatzidis H.	- Nephrological Center, University of Athens, Aretaion University Hospital, Athens, Greece.

APPENDIX II

COMPANIES AND INSTITUTIONS MENTIONED IN THIS REPORT

COMPANIES

ABG-SEMCA, S.A.
3, Villa Thoréton
B.P. N° 502
75725 Paris Cedex 15
France

AKZO N.V.
Postbus 186
Ijssellaan 82
Arnhem
The Netherlands

AMERICAN MEDICAL PRODUCTS CORP.
P.O. Drawer 190
Freehold, New Jersey 0772
U.S.A.

AMICON CORPORATION
25 Hartwell Avenue
Lexington, Massachussetts 02173
U.S.A.

ASAHI MEDICA CO. LTD
Hibiya-Mitsui Building
1-2, Yarakucho 1-Chome
Chiyoda-Ku
Tokyo

AVON MEDICALS LTD.
1649 Perschore Road
Stircheley
Birmingham B30 3DR
England

C.R. BARD, INC.
731 Central Avenue
Murray Hill, New Jersey 07974
U.S.A.

BELLCO S.p.A.
P.O. Box 92
41037 Mirandola (Modena)
Italy

B. BRAUN MELSUNGEN AG
Postfach 110 and 120
3508 Melsungen
West Germany

COBE LABORATORIES, INC.
1202 Oak Street
Lakewood, Colorado 80215
U.S.A.

CORDIS DOW CORPORATION
999 Brickel Avenue
P.O. Box 450990
Miami, Florida 33145
U.S.A.

DASCO
Via C. Battisti 3
41037 Mirandola (Modena)
Italy

DIDECO S.p.A.
P.O. Box 87
41037 Mirandola (Modena)
Italy

DRAKE WILLOCH
Subsidiary of BECTON, DICKINSON AND COMPANY
13520 S.E. Pheasant Court
Portland, Oregon 97222
U.S.A.

THE DYLADE COMPANY LTD.
45 Brindley Road
Astmoor Industrial Estate
Runcorn
Cheshire
England

ENKA AG
P.O. 200916
D5600 Wuppertal 2
West Germany

EXTRACORPOREAL AND MEDICAL SPECIALTIES, INC.
Royal and Ross Roads
King of Prussia, Pennsylvania 19406
U.S.A.

DR. E. FRESENIUS KG
Dietigheimerstrasse 1-3
Postfach 1480
6380 Bad Homburg v.d.H.
West Germany

GAMBRO AB
Magistratsvägen 16
220 Lund 10
Sweden

HAEMONETICS
400 Woodroad
Braintree, M
U.S.A.

HOSPAL
7, avenue Lionel-Terray
69330 Meyzieu
France

IBM
P.O. Box
Princeton, New Jersey 08540
U.S.A.

MELTEC LTD.
Station Approach
Bourne End
Berkhamsted
Hertfordshire
England

A/S NYCOTRON
P.O. Box 425
3001 Drammen
Norway

ORGANON TEKNIKA BV
Industrielaan 84
5349 AG Oss
The Netherlands

PARKER BIOMEDICAL
17352 Von Karman Av.
Irvine, California 92714
U.S.A.

RHONE-POULENC, S.A.
23, avenue Franklin D. Roosevelt
75008 Paris
France

SANDOZ AG
Holeestrasse 87
4015 Basel
Switzerland

SORIN BIOMEDICA, S.p.A.
13040 Saluggia
Italy

TORAI
2-2 Nihonbashi-Muromachi
Chuoku
Tokyo
Japan

TRAVENOL LABORATORIES, INC.
1 Baxter Parkway
Deerfield, Illinois 60015
U.S.A.

INSTITUTIONS

ANED (Italian Association for Haemodialysed Patients)
Piazza San Fedele, 4
20121 Milano
Italy

EUROTRANSPLANT FOUNDATION,
c/o Bloodbank,
University Hospital,
Rijnsburgerweg 10,
2333 AA - Leiden,
The Netherlands

FRANCETRANSPLANT,
Laboratoire d'Immuno-haematologie,
Hopital Saint-Lous,
2 Place du Dr. Fournier,
75010 Paris
France

SCANDIATRANSPLANT,
Tissue Typing Laboratory,
Aarhus Kommunehospital,
DK 800 AARHUS C.,
Denmark

SUISSE-TRANSPLANT,
Unite d'Immunologie de Transplantation,
Hopital Cantonal,
Rue Micheli du Crest 24
1211 Geneve 4,
Switzerland

UK TRANSPLANT SERVICE
Southmead Road
Bristol BS10 5ND
United Kingdom

AKNOWLEDGMENTS

The authors wish to thank the following people for the help received for the preparation of this report.

Dr. O. Akerblon
Darolinska Hospital
Blood Center
Stockholm
Sweden

Dr. M. Asaba
Huddige Hospital
Renal Medicine
Stockholm
Sweden

Dr. Borini
Organon Teknika
Roma
Italy

Dr. D. Brancaccio
Osp. San Paolo
Milano
Italy

Prof. C. Casciani
Pat. Chirurg. V
Università di Roma
Roma
Italy

Dr. Casolino
Consiglio Nazionale delle Ricerche
Roma
Italy

Dr. E. Denti
Sorin Biomedica
Saluggia
Italy

Prof. L. Donato
Università di Pisa
Pisa
Italy

Dr. Francois
Dir. Général
Administration de la Medicine Sociale
Bruxelles
Belgium

Dr. H.J. Gurland
Medizinische Klinik
Universität München
West Germany

Dr. Levaux
Secr. Général du
Fond de la Recherche Scientific Médicale
Bruxelles
Belgium

Mr. B. Longfellow
Dept. Health and Social Security
London WCIB - 5ED
United Kingdom

Ing. A. Musso
ADAD
Genova
Italy

Dr. P. Olsson
Karolinska Hospital
Dept. Exp. Surgery
Stockholm
Sweden

Dr. E. Petrella
Bellco S.p.A.
Mirandola (MO)
Italy

Dr. Rocchi
Consiglio Nazionale delle Ricerche
Roma
Italy

Mrs. U. Takman
National Board of Health and Welfare
Stockholm
Sweden

Dr. J.L. Vanherweghem
Hopital Erasme
Service de Nephrologie et de Chirurgie
Bruxelles
Belgium

Dr. A.J. Wing
St. Thomas Hospital
London SE 1 7EH
United Kingdom

BLOOD DETOXIFICATION AS A THERAPEUTIC TECHNIQUE

PROBLEMS AND PERSPECTIVES

L I T E R A T U R E

PAPERS

Dialysis and Blood/Material Interaction

Alfrey A.C., Smythe W.R., Trace metals and regular dialysis. in Replacement of Renal Function by Dialysis. W. Drukker, F.M. Parson, J.F. Maher eds., Martinus Nijhoff, The Hague, 1978, p. 647.

Asaba H., Fürst, P., Oulés R., Yahiel V., Zimmermann L., Bergström J. The effect of hemodialysis on endogenous middle molecules in uremic patients. Clin Nephrol., 11 (5): 257, 1979.

Avram M.M., Feinfeld, D.A., Gau A.C. Non A - non B hepatitis: a new syndrome in uraemic patients. Proc. Eur. Dial. Transpl. Assoc. 16: 141, 1979.

Babb A.L., Popovich R.P., Christopher T.G. et al. The genesis of the square meter-hour hypothesis. Trans. Am. Soc. Artif. Intern. Organs. 17: 81, 1971.

Babb A.L., Farrel P.C., Uvelli, D.A. et al., Haemodialyser evaluation by examination of solute molecular spectra. Trans. Am. Soc. Artif. Intern. Organ 18: 98, 1972.

Bagdade J., Casaretto A., Albers J., Effect of chronic uremia, haemodialysis and renal transplantation on plasma lipids and lipoprotein in man. J. Lab. Clin. Med. 87: 37, 1976.

Baker L.D.Jr., Johnson J.M., Goldfarb D. Expanded polytetrafluoroethylene (PTFE) subcutaneous arteriovenous conduit: an improved vascular access for chronic haemodialysis. Trans. Am. Soc. Artif. Intern. Organs 22:382, 1976.

Ball, J.H. Bukkus D.E., Madison D.S. Effect of subtotal parathyroidectomy on dialysis dementia. Nephron 18: 151, 1977.

Bergström J., Asaba H., Fürst P., Oulés R. Dialysis ultrafiltration and blood pressure.
Proc. Eur. Dial. Transplant Assoc. 13: 293, 1976.

Bergström J. Ultrafiltration without dialysis for removal of fluid and solutes in uremia.
Clin. Nephrol. 9: 156, 1978.

Bergström J., Fürst P., Uremic toxins. Replacement of renal function by dialysis. Ed. by W. Drukker, F.M. Parson, J.F. Maher,, The Hague, Martinus Nijhoff, 335, 1978.

Blumenkrantz M.J., Gahl G.M., Kopple J.D., Kamdar A.V., Jones M.R., Kessel, M., Coburn J.W. Protein losses during peritoneal dialysis.
Kidney Int. 19: 593, 1981.

Borges, N., Fryd D., Rosa A. et al., Acetate versus bicarbonate in acute haemodialysis.
Clin. Res. 27: 410 A, 1979.

Brancaccio D., Damasso R., Spinuler H., Sterzi R., Vallar G., Neuropsychological performances of patients dialysed for more than 10 years. in Uremia - Pathobiology of Patients treated for 10 years or more.
C. Giordano, E.A. Friedman eds., Wichtig Ed., Milan, 1981, p. 126

* Brescia, M.J., Cimino J.E., Appel K. et al. Chronic hemodialysis using venipuncture and a surgically created fistula.
N. Engl. J. Med. 275: 1089, 1966.

Brunner F.P., Brynger H., Chantle C., Donckerwolcke R.A., Hathway R.A., Jacobs C., Selwood N.H., Wing A.J., Combined report on regular dialysis and transplantation in Europe

*See pag. 15

IX, 1978.
Proc. Eur. Dial. Transplant. Assoc. 15: 3, 1978.

Burton B.T., Hirschman G.H., Treatment trends of end stage renal disease in the United States.
Proc. 2nd Meet. Int. Soc. Artif. Intern. Organs. 29, 1979.

Butt K.M.H. , Friedman E.A., Kountz S.L. Angioacces Curr. Probl. Surg. 13(9): 1, 1976.

Brynger H., Brunner F.P., Chantler C., Donckerwolke R.A. Jacobs C., Kramer P., Selwood N.H., Wing A.J.
Combined report on regular dialysis and transplantation in Europe, X, 1979.
Proc.Eur. Dial. Transplant Ass. 17: 2, 1980.

Cambi U., Dall'Aglio P., Savazzi G., Arisi L., Rossi E., Migone L. Clinical assessment of haemodialysis patients with reduced small molecules removal.
Proc. Eur. Dial. Transpl. Assoc. 9: 67, 1972.

Cavagna R., Casal D., De Paoli Vitali E., Tessarin C., Badiani G., Camaiore E., Nicolini M.A., Perotta V. Interchangeable abdominal catheter for peritoneal dialysis.
Int. J. Artific. Organs 4: 108, 1981.

Coburn J.W., Llach F., Renal osteodystrophy and maintenance dialysis, in Replacement of Renal Function by Dialysis W. Drukker, F.M. Parson, J.F. Maher eds., Martinus Nijhoff, The Hague, 1978, p. 571.

Cole J.J. Quinton W.E., Williams C., Murray J.S., Sherris J.C., The pumpless low temperature haemodialysis system.
Trans. Am. Soc. Artif. Intern. Organs 8: 209, 1962.

Coursaget P., Maupas P., Dubois F., Duncker J., Caudeau A. Hépatite non A - non B chez six malades hemodyalisé. Nouv. Presse Med. 7: 3515, 1978.

Crosnier J., Jungers P., Couroneé A.M., Laplance A., Benhanon E., Degos F., Lacour B., Prunet P., Cerisier Y., and Guesry P., Randomised Placebo - controlled trial of Hepatitis B surface antigen vaccine in french haemodialysis Units: I, Medical staff. Lancet I, 454, 1981.

Crosnier J., Jungers P., Couroncé A.M., Laplance A., Benhanon E., Degos F., Lacour B., Prunet P., Cerisier Y., and Guesry P. Randomised Placebo - controlled trial of hepatitis B surface antigen vaccin in french haemodialysis units: II, Haemodialysis patients. Lancet I, 797, 1981.

Diaz-Duxo J.A., Walker P.J., Farmer C.A., Chandler J.T., Holt K.L. Continuous cycling peritoneal dialysis (CCPD) (abstract) Am. Soc. Nephrol. 13: 38A, 1980.

Drukker W., Person F.M., Gordon A., Practical applications of dialysate regeneration: the Redy system in replacement of renal function by dialysis. Ed. by W. Drukker, F.M. Person, J.F. Maher, The Hague, Martinus Nijhoff, 1978, 244.

Falb R.D., Leininger R.I., Grode G., Crowley J., Surface-bound heparin. Adv. Exp. Med. Biol. 52: 365, 1974.

Friedman, E.A., Delano B.G., Can the world afford uremia therapy? Proc. 8th Int. Congr. Nephrol., 577, 1981.

Galbraith R.M., Dienstag J.L., Purcell R.N., Gower P.H., Zuckerman A.J., Williams, R. Non A - Non B hepatitis associated with chronic liver disease in a haemodialysis unit.
Lancet I., 951, 1979.

Giordano C., Esposito R., Pluvio M. An improved oxystarch in the treatment of renal failure. In Artificial Organs Proc. 2nd Strathclyde Bioengineering Seminar. The Macmillan Press Ltd., 1977, p. 327.

Giordano C., Esposito R., Di Leo V.A., Pluvio M. Oxycellulose as oral sorbent in uremia.
Clin. Nephrol. 11: 142, 1979.

Giordano C. Sorbents and their clinical applications. Academic Press, New York, 1980.

Giordano C., Prolongation of survival for a decade or more by low protein diet, in Uremia. Pathobiology of patients treated for 10 year or more. C. Giordano, E.A. Friedman eds., Wichtig Ed., Milan, 1981, p. 4.

Gotloib L., Servadio C., Ascites in patients undergoing maintenance haemodialysis: report of six cases and physiopathologic approach.
Am. J. Med. 61: 465, 1976.

Gott V.L., Wall-bound heparin. Historical background and current clinical applications.
Adv. Exp. Med. Biol. 52: 351, 1974.

Graefe U., Milutinovich., Follette W.C., Vizzo J.E., Babb A.L., Schribner B.H. Less dialysis-induced morbidity and vascular instability with bicarbonate in dialysate.
Ann. Intern. Med. 88: 332, 1978

Griffin J.H., Cochrane C.G. Mechanism for the involvement of high molecular weight kininogen in surface dependent reactions of Hageman factor.
Proc. Natl. Acad. Sci. USA 73: 2554, 1976.

Guarnieri G., Faccini L., Lipartiti T., Ranieri F., Spangaro F., Giuntini D., Toigo G., Dardi F. Berguier-Vidali F., Raimondi A., Simple method for nutritional assessment in hemodialysed patients.
Am. J. Clin. Nutr. 33: 1598, 1980.

Gupta S.K., Weith F.J., Three year experience with expanded polytetrafluoroethylene arterial graft for limb salvage.
Am. J. Surg. 140: 214, 1980.

Gurland H.J., Brunner F.P., Chantler C., Jacobs C., Scharer K., Selwood N.H., Spies G., Wing A.J., Combined report on regular dialysis and transplantation in Europe VI, 1975.
Proc. Eur. Dial. Transplant. Assoc. 13: 3, 1976.

Gurland H.J. Did the Federal Republic of Germany attain that degree of uremia therapy that may be expected from it on the basis of its gross national product.
Proc. Second Congress Intern. Soc. Artif. Organs 9, 1979.

Gurland H.J., Wing A.J., Jacobs C., Brunner F.P., Comparative review between dialysis and transplantation in replacement of renal function by dialysis. W. Drukker, F.M. Parson, J.F. Maher eds., Martinous Nijhoff, The Hague 1978, p. 663.

Haire H., Sherrard D., Scardapani D. Cardiovascular risk factors in dialysis patients.
Am. Soc. Artif. Intern. Organs 5: 33, 1976.

Hall P.W., Doichinov D., Dinev J., Dimitrov Ts., Radovanovic Z., Dammin G., Balkan Nephropathy:

Relationship with transitional cell cancer.
Proc. 8th Int. Congr. Nephrol. 1210, 1981.

Heidland A., Kult J., Rockel A., Heidbredler E. Evaluation of essential amino acids and keto acids in uremic patients on low protein diet.
Am. J. Clin. Nutr. 31: 1784, 1978.

Hegstrom R.M., Murray J.S., Pendras J.P. et al., Haemodialysis in the treatment of chronic uremia.
Trans. Am. Soc. Artif. Intern. Organs 7: 136, 1961.

Jacobs C., Broyer, M., Brunner F.P., Brynger H., Douckerwolcke R.A., Kramer P., Selwood, Wing A.J. Talk manuscript and figures from combined report on intermittent dialysis and renal transplantation in Europe, XI, 1980.
18th Congress Eur. Dial. Transplant Ass., 1981.

Jeekel J., Van der Linden C.J., Vegt P.A. Bunrman W.A., Harder F., and Persijn G. Modification of Kidney graft survival in dog and man by pre - operative transfusion to the donor.
Proc. Eur. Dial. Transpl. Assoc. 17, 457, 1980.

Jozefowicz M., Jozefowicz J., Fougnot C., Labarre D., Heparin-like insoluble biomaterials (Abstract)
Proc. 27th Int. Symp. Macromol., 1314, 1981.

Kanna R., Oroupoulus D.G., Dombros N. et al. The present state of continuous ambulatory peritoneal dialysis (CAPD).
Peritoneal Dial. Bull.(Toronto Western Hospital) 1, 1981 (in press).

Kataoka K., Tsuruta T., Biomedical behaviour of synthetic polyion complexes toward blood platelets. Makromol. Chem. 181: 1363, 1980.

Kiil F., Development of a parallel flow artificial kidney in plastics.
Acta Chir. Scand. (Suppl.) 253: 142, 1960.

Kim S.W., Ebert C.D., Mc Rea J.C., Pharmacological modification of polymers for the enhancement of blood compatibility (abstract)
Proc. 3rd Meeting Int. Soc. Artif. Organs, 1981.

Kjellstrand C.M. Current problems in long-term haemodialysis.
Dial. Transpl. 9 (4) : 295, 1980.

Kjellstrand C.M. Hemodialysis. The gold standard.
Proc. 8th Int. Congr. Neph. 708, 1981.

Klein E., Progress in haemodialysis and membranes. The last 20 years.
Clin. Nephrol. 9, 131, 1978.

Knochel J.P., Endocrine changes in patients on chronic dialysis , in Replacement of renal function by dialysis, W Drukker, F.M. Parsons, J.F. Maher, eds., Martinus Nijhoff, The Hague. 1978, p. 546.

Koch K.M., Frei U., Fassbinder W., Haemolysis and anemia in anti N-like antibody positive haemodialysis patients.
Trans. Am. Soc. Artif. Intern. Organs, 24: 709, 1978.

Larsson R., Eriksson J.C., Largergren M., Olsson P.
Platelet and plasma coagulation coagulability of heparinized and sulphated surfaces.
Thrombos. Res., 15: 157, 1979.

Lee H.A., Talbot S., Rowlands A., Jackson M.A., Dietary management of chronic renal failure with oral amino acids.
Nutr.Metab. 24: 50, 1980.

Lee H.A., Jackson M.A., Keto acid therapy in chronic renal failure patients on moderately protein restricted diets in Uremia. Pathobiology of patients treated for 10 years or more, C. Giordano, E.A. Friedman eds., Wichtig Ed., Milan, 1981, p. 8.

Lewis L.M., Flechtner T.W., Kerkay J., et al., Bis (2-ethylhexyl) phtalate concentration in the serum of haemodialysis patients.
Clin. Chem. 24: 741, 1978.

Lindner A., Charra B., Sherrad D.J., Scribner B.H., Accelerated atherosclerosis in prolonged maintenance hemodialysis
N. Engl. J. Med. 290: 697, 1974.

Lyman D.J., New progress in biomedical polymer materials.
Pure Appl. Chem. 50: 427, 1978.

Maiorca R., Castellani A., Mingozzi G., Panzetta G.O., Usberti M. Short time personalized: good results in spite of high levels of small and middle molecules.
Proc. Eur. Dial. Transpl. Assoc. 11: 146, 1974.

Man N.K., Terlain B., Paris J., Werner G., Sausse A., Funk-Brentano J.L., An approach to "middle molecules" identification in artificial kidney dialysate, with reference to neuropathy prevention.
Trans. Am. Soc. Artif. Intern. Organs 19:320, 1973.

Manis T., Friedman E.A. Dialytic therapy for irreversible uremia.
N. Engl. J. Med. 301: 1260, 1979.

Marconi W., Bartoli F., Mantovani E., Pittalis F., Settembri L., Cordova C., Musca A., Alessandri C., Development of new antithrombogenic surfaces by employing platelet antiaggregating agents: preparation and characterization. Trans. Am. Soc. Artif. Intern. Organs, 25: 280, 1979.

Mason R.G., Zucker W.H., Bilinsky R.T., Shinoda B.A., Mohammed S.F. Blood components on used and reused dialysis membranes. Biomater Med. Devices. Artif. Organs 1977.

Massry S.G., Malluche H.H., Goldstein D.A., Schoeppe W., Influence of long-term haemodialysis on uremic bone disease, in Chemio-pathobiology of patients treated for 10 year or more. C. Giordano, E.A. Friedman Ed. Wichtig Editore, Milan, 1981, p. 73.

Mc Rea J.C., Kim S.W. Characterization of controlled release of prostaglandin from polymer matrices for thrombus prevention. Trans. Am. Soc. Artif. Intern. Organs, 25: 746, 1978.

Mery J.P., Simon N., Couroncé A.M. Hépatite chez le hemodyalisés chroniques, 5 observations. Nouv. Presse Med. 8: 3973, 1979.

Mirahmadi K.S., Kay J.H., Miller J.H., Gonenau J.T., Rosens M., Clinical evaluation of patients dialysed with double Gambro 4 hours, three times per week. Proc. Eur. Dial. Transpl. Assoc. 11: 121, 1974.

Mohammad S.F., Whitworth C., Chuang H.Y.K., Lundblad R.L., Mason R.G., Multiple active forms of thrombin binding to platelets and effects on platelet function. Proc. Natl. Acad. Sci. USA 73: 1660, 1976.

Mohammad S.F., Hardison M.D., Glem C.H., Morton B.D., Bolan J.C., Mason R.G., Adhesion of human blood plate-

lets to glass on polymer surface I. Studies with platelets in plasma.
Haemostasis 3: 257, 1974.

Nakagawa S., Multifactorial evaluation of haemofiltration therapy in comparison with conventional haemodialysis.
Artif. Organs 4: 94, 1980.

Neegaard J., Nielsen B., Faurby V. et al., On the exudation of platicizers from PVC haemodialysis tubing.
Nephron 14: 263, 1975.

Nylas E., Ward S.R. Jr. Development of blood compatible elastomers. V. Surface structure and blood compatibility of Avcothane elastomers.
J. Biomed. Mater. Res. Symp. 8: 69, 1977.

Ogden D.A., Kopec G., Gui A.D. Cost effectiveness of multiple dialyzer use.
Dial Transplant. 10(5): 407, 1981.

Opelz G., Terasaki P.I., Graver B. et al. Correlation between number of pretransplant blood transfusion and kidney graft survival. Transplant Proc. 11: 145, 1979.

Oreopoulos D.G., Robson M., Izatt S., Clayton S., de Veber G.A. A simple and safe technique for continuous ambulatory peritoneal dialysis.
Trans. Am. Soc. Artif. Intern. Organs 24: 484, 1978.

Ota K., Development and present status of chronic dialysis and kidney transplantation in Japan.
Trans. Int. Soc. Artif. Intern. Organs. 21, 1979.

Parkinson I.S., Ward M.K., Feest T.G. Fracturing osteodystrophy and dialysis encepholopathy Lancet II: 406, 1979.

Pendras J.P., Cole J.J., Tu T.H., Scribner B.H. Improved tech nique of continuous flow hemodialysis.
Trans. Am. Soc. Artif. Intern. Organs 7: 27, 1961.

Pierides A.M., Ward M.K., Kerr D.N.S., Haemodialysis encephalopathy: Possible role of phosphate depletion.
Lancet II, 1234, 1976.

Popovic R.P., Monerief J.W., Decherd J.F., Bomar J.B., Pyle W.B. The definition of a novel portable/wearable equilibrium pe ritoneal dialysis technique (abstract).
Trans Am. Soc. Artif. Int. Organs 5: 64, 1976.

Prince A.M., Szmuness W., Mann M.K., et al., Hepatitis B immunoglobulin: final report of a controlled multicenter trial efficacy in prevention of dialysis hepatitis.
J. Infect. Dis. 137: 131, 1978.

Quellhorst E., Schuenemann B., Borgard J., Influence of hemofil tration on blood pressure regulation.
Clin. Nephrol., 11: 150, 1979.

Richards V., Hobbs C., Murray T., Muller J., Incidence and sequelae of malnutrition (NNUT) in chronic haemodialysis (HD) patients.
Kidney Internat. 14: 683, 1978.

Shiffan S., Lee P., Partial purification and characterization of contact activator cofactor.
J. Clin. Invest. 56: 1082, 1975.

Schmer G. The biological activity of covalently immobilized he parin.
Trans. Am. Soc. Artif. Intern. Organs. 18: 321, 1972.

Setäla K., Heinonen H., Schreck-Purola. Uremic waste recovery: in vitro studies.
Proc. Eur. Dial. Transplant. Assoc. 9: 514, 1972.

Setäla K., Bacterial enzymes in uremia management.
Kidney Int. 13: 194, 1978.

Shaldon S., Progress in dialysis and the problems of patient tolerance to treatment. Introduction.
Proc. 8th Int. Congr. Nephrol. Athens 1981, 689.

Shinaberger, J.H., Miller J.H., Rosenblatt M.G., Gardner P.W., Carpenter G.W., Martin F.E., Clinical studies of low flow dialysis with membrane highly permeable to middle weight molecules.
Trans. Am. Soc. Artif. Intern. Organs. 18: 82, 1972.

Singh S., Mitra S., Berman L.B., Ascites in patients on mainte nance haemodialysis.
Nephron 12: 114, 1974.

Slatopolsky E., Gray R., Adams N.D., Lewis J., Hruska K., Martin K., Klahr S., De Luca H., Leman J., The pathogenesis of secondary hyperparathyroidism in early renal failure, in Vi tamin D. Basic research and its clinical applications. A.W. Normal, K. Schefer, D.V. Herrath, H.G. Grigoleit, J.W. Coburn, H.F. De Luca, E.B. Mawer, T. Suda, Eds. Walter De Gruyter, Berlin and New York, 1979, p. 1209.

Snidman D.R., Bryan J.A., Dixon R.E., Prevention of nosocomial viral hepatitis, type B (hepatitis B).
Ann. Intern. Med. 83: 838, 1975.

Sorm M., Nespurek S., Mrkvickova L., Kalal J., Vorlova Z., Anti coagulation activity of some sulfate-containing polymers of the methacrylate type.
J. Polym. Sci., Polym. Symp. 66: 349, 1979.

Sugitachi A., Takagi K. Antithrombogenicity of immobilized uro kinase. Clinical application.
Int. J. Artif. Organs, 1(2): 88, 1978.

Szmuness W., Stevens, C.E., Harley E.J., Zang E.A., Oleszko W.R., William D.C., Sadovsky R., Morrison J.M. and Kellner A. Hepatitis B racine. Demonstration of efficacy in a controlled clinical trial in a high-risk population in the United States.
N. Engl. J. Med., 303(15), 833, 1980.

Taclob L., Needle M., Drug-induced encephalopathy in patients on maintenance haemodialysis.
Lancet II, 404, 1976.

Teschan P.E., Giun H.E., Bourne J.R., Walker P.J., Ward J.W. Quantitative neurobehavioral responses to renal failure and maintenance dialysis.
Trans. Am. Soc. Artif. Intern. Organs 21: 488, 1975.

Thomas F.T., Lee H.M., Factors in the differential rate of arteriosclerosis (AS) between long surviving renal transplant recipients and dialysis patients.
Ann. Surg. 184: 342, 1976.

Vanherweghem J.L. Private communication, 1981.

Vroman L., Adams A.L., Klings M., Interaction among human blood protein and interfaces.
Fed. Proc. 30: 1494, 1971.

Wehle B., Asaba H., Castenfors J., Fürst P., Grahn A., Cunnarson B., Shaldon D., Bergstrom J., The influence of dialysis fluid composition on blood pressure response during dialysis.
Clin. Nephrol. 10: 62, 1978.

Winchester J.F., Clinical application of haemoperfusion in uremia. In Artificial Organs. Proceedings of 2nd Stratchclyde Bioengineering Seminar. The Mcmillan Press Ltd. 1977, p. 188.

Wing A.J., Brunner F.P., Brynger H., Chantler C., Douckerwolcke R.A., Gurland H.J., Jacobos C., Kramer P., and Selwood N.H. Dialysis Dementia in Europe. Report from the Registration Commitee of the European Dialysis and Transplantation Association.
Lancet II, 190, 1980.

Yatzidis H., Knotzicos D., Digenis P. Newer oral sorbents in uremia.
Clin. Nephrol. 11: 105, 1979.

Yatzidis H., Knotzicos D., Digenis P., Oral locust bean gum therapy of uremia. Favorable effect on biological abnormalities and hypertension.
Dial. Transplant. 9(4): 313, 1980.

Young T.K. Current status of intestinal lavage.
Int. J. Artif. Organs, 2: 11, 1979.

Plasmapheresis

Abell C.W., Hodgins D.S., Stith W.J. An in vivo evaluation of the chemotherapeutic potency of phenylalanine ammonia-lyase. Canc. Res. 33: 2529, 1973.

Adriaenssens K., Karcher D., Lowenthal A., Therheggen H.G. Use of enzyme - loaded erythrocytes in familial hyperargininaemia. Clin. Chem. 23: 323, 1976.

Agishi T., Kaneko I., Hasuo Y., Sanaka T., Ota K., Amemiya H., Sugino N., Double filtration plasmapheresis with no or minimal amount of blood derivative for substitution, in Plasma Exchange. Proc. Int. Symp. Cologne, 6th and 7th June 1980. H.G. Sieberth ed. Stuttgart, N.Y.: Schattaner, 1980 p. 53.

Asanuma, Y., Smith J.W., Suwa S., Zawicki J., Nosè Y. Membrane plasmapheresis: platelet and protein effects on filtration. Proc. Eur. Soc. Trans. Ass. 6: 308, 1979.

Asanuma Y., Malchesky P.S., Zawiscky I., Smith J.W., Carey W.D., Ferguson D.R., Hermann R.E., Nosè Y. Clinical hepatic support by on-line plasma treatment with multiple sorbents: evaluation of system performance. Trans. Am. Soc. Artif. Intern. Organs. 26: 400, 1980.

Bach J. F. Principes de Thèrapeutique immunologique éléments pour une nouvelle stratégie. Revue de Praticien 38: 895, 1980.

Baker R.E., Jefferson L.S., and Shiman R. Immunocytochemical identification of phenylalanine hydroxylase and albumin in cultured hepatoma cells and isolated rat hepatocytes. J. Cell Biol., 90: 145, 1981.

Bansal S.C., Bansal B.R., Thomas H.L., Siegel P.D., Rhoads J.E., Cooper D.R., Terman D.S., Mark R. Ex vivo removal of serum Igg in a patient with colon carcinoma.
Cancer 42: 1, 1978.

Benbunam M., Bussel A., Reviron J., Boiron M., Bernard J.J. Les trasfusion de granulocytes normaux prélevé sur separateur de cellules. Resultats techniques et cliniques.
Nouv. Rev. Franc. Hemat. 13: 469, 1973.

Besinger W.I., Baker D.A., Buckner C.D., Clift R.A., Thomas E.A. Immunoadsorption for removal of A and B blood-group antibodies.
New Engl. J. Med. 304: 160, 1981.

Billah M.M., Finean J.B., Coleman R., Mitchell R.H. Permeability characteristics of erythrocyte ghosts prepared under isoionic conditions by a glycol-induced osmotic lysis.
Biochim Biophys. ACTA 465: 515, 1977.

Briggs W.A., Johnson J.P., Telchman S., Yeager H.C., Wilson C.B. Antiglomerular basement membrane antibody-mediated glomerulonephritis and Goodasture's syndrome.
Medicine 58: 34, 1978.

Burgs aler E.A., Pineda A.A., Ellefson R.D. Removal of plasma lipoproteins from circulating blood with a heparin-agarose column.
Mayo Clinic Proc. 55: 180, 1980.

Callegaro L., Barbieri U., Denti E. Selective detoxification: hemoperfusion on antiphenobarbital antibody immobilized on solid phase (abstract).
Trans. Am. Soc. Artif. Intern. Organs 10: 40, 1981.

Callegaro L., Boniolo A., Malinverni A. Immobilization of ligandin on hollow fiber reactors.
Int. Symp. Artif. Liver Support. (abstract), Celle (W. Germany), 1980.

Cederbaum S.D., Shaw K.N.F., Spector E.B., Verity M.A., Snodgrass P.J., Sugarman G.I. Hyperargininaemia with arginase deficiency.
Pediat. Res. 13: 827, 1979.

Chalopin J.M. Rifle G., Tune J.M., Cortet P., Severac M. Immunological finding during successful treatment of HBs Ag - associated polyartheritis nodosa by plasmapheresis alone.
Brit. Med. J. 280: 368, 1980.

Chang T.M.S., Artificial cells: The use of hybrid systems.
Artif. Organs 4: 264, 1980.

Chang T.M.S. Encapsulation of enzymes, cell contents, cell, vaccines, antigens, antiserum, cofactors, hormones and proteins. In Biomedical Application of Immobilized Enzymes and Proteins Vol. 1, T.M.S. Chang ed. Plenum Press 1977, p. 69.

Chang T.M.S. The in vivo effects of semipermeable microcapsules containing L-asparaginase on 6C3HED lynphosarcoma.
Nature, 229: 117, 1971.

Chang T.M.S., Malouf C., Resurreccion E. Artificial cells containing multienzyme system for the sequential conversion of urea into ammonia glutammate, and alanine.
Proc. 2nd Meet. Int. Soc. Artif. Organs. 284, 1979.

Chopek M., McCullough J.J. Some hematologic and biochemical effect of plasma exchange (abstract).
Transfusion 19: 651, 1979.

Currie G.A., Basham C. Differential arginine dependence and the selective cytotoxic effect of activated macrophages for malignant cells in vitro.
Br. J. Cancer 38: 653 1978a.

Dan P.C., Petajan J.H., Johnson K.P., Panitch H.S., and Borustein M.B. Plasmapheresis in multiple sclerosis: Preliminary findings.
Neurology 30: 1023, 1980.

Denti E., Freston J.W., Marciosio M., Kolff W.J., Toward a bioartificial drug metabolizing system: gel immobilized liver cell microsomes.
Trans. Am. Soc. Artif. Intern. Organs. 22: 693, 1976.

Fritz R.R., Hodgins D.S., and Abell C.W. Phenylalanine ammonia-lyase. Introduction and purification from past and clearance in mammals.
J. Biol. Chem. 251, 4646, 1976.

Garland R.C., and Cori C.F. Protein synthesis with membrane - bound polysomes and albumin messenger RNA from livers of mutant mice.
Mol. Cellular Biochem. 36: 29, 1981.

Gurland H.J., Heinze Y., Lee H.A. Topics in therapeutic plasma exchange: classification of published work. In Therapeutic Plasma Exchange. H.J. Gurland, V. Heize, H.A. Lee eds. Springer, Berlin, Neidelberg, New York 1981, p. 203.

Gurland H.J., Samtleben W., Blumenstein M., Randerson D.H., Schmidt B. Clinical applications of macromolecular separations.
Proc. Am. Soc. Artif. Intern. Organs 27: 0004, 1981 (in press).

Higly D.J., Henderson E.S. Granulocyte transfusion therapy. Ann. Rev. Med. 26: 289, 1975.

Hydén H. Enzyme therapy and immuno-adsorption by an extracorporeal device.
Biomat. Med. Dev. Artif. Organs 8: 1, 1980.

Hollàn S.R. Clinical significance of circulating immune complexes: Effect of plasmapheresis.
Haematologia 12: 69, 1978/79.

Isbister J.P. Plasma exchange: a selective form of blood-letting. Med. J. Austr. 2: 167, 1979.

Jackson J.A., Halvorson H.R., Fulrong J.W., Lucast K.D., Shone J.D. A new extracorporeal reactor - dialyzer for enzyme therapy using immobilized L-asparaginase.
J. Pharm. Exp. Ther. 209: 271, 1980.

Jones J.V., Bucknall R.C., Cumming R.H. et al. Plasmapheresis in the management of acute systemic lupus erythematosus.
Lancet I, 709, 1976.

Lauterburg B.H., Pineda A.A., Burgstaler E.A., Taswell H.F., Dickson E.R., Carlson G.L. Treatment of pruritus of cholestasis by plasma perfusion through USP-charcoal - coated glass beads.
Lancet II, 53, 1980.

Malchesky P.S., Asanuma Y., Smith J., Zawicky I., Nosè Y. Membrane plasmapheresis with on-line plasma treatment. In Hemoperfusion Parts 1. S. Sideman, T.M.S. Chang eds.
Hemisphere Publ. Comp., Washington 1980, p. 111.

Malchesky P.S., Asanuma Y., Zawicki I. Blumenstein M., Calabrese L., Kyo A., Krakaner R., Nosé Y. On line separation of macromolecules by membrane filtration with cryogenation.
Artif. Organs. 4: 205, 1980.

Newsom-Davis J., Pinching A.J., Vincent A., Wilson S.G. Function of circulating antibody to acetilcholine receptor in myastenia gravis: Investigation by plasma exchance.
Neurology, 28: 266, 1978.

Ouchi K., Piatkiewicz W., Malchensky P.S., Herman R., Nosè Y. An efficient, specific and blood compatible sorbent system for hepatic assist.
Trans. Am. Soc. Artif. Inter. Organs 24: 246, 1978.

Peterson J.A. Clonal variation in albumin messanger RNA activity in hepatoma cells.
Proc. Nat. Acad. Sci. USA 73: 2056, 1976.

Pineda A.A. Therapeutic plasmapheresis: New technics and applications in therapeutic hemapheresis: A technical Workshop. Berkman E.M., Unlas J. eds.
American Association of Blood Banks, Washington, D.C. 1980 p. 139.

Raich P.C., Traver M.I. Therapeutic plasmapheresis.
Wis. Med. J. 78: 37, 1979.

Ravindranat Y. Intermittent intrathecal methotrexate and fractional radiation plus chemotherapy in acute lymphoblastic leukaemia.
Astr. Int. Ped. Oncol. Conf. (in press), Rome, Oct. 22-24, 1981.

Ray P.K., Besa E., Idiculla A., Rhoads J.E., Basset J.G., Cooper D.R. Efficient removal of abnormal immunoglobulin G from the plasma of a multiple myeloma patient; description of a new method for treatment of the hyperviscosity syndrome.
Cancer 45: 2633, 1980.

Ray P.K., Besa E., Idiculla A., Rhoads J.E., Basset J.G. Cooper D.R. Extracorporeal immunoadsorption of myeloma Igg and autoimmune antibodies - a clinically feasible modality of treatment.
Clin. Exper. Immunol. 42: 308, 1980.

Reed W.P., Williams R.C. Immune complexes in infection diseases.
Adv. Int. Med. 22: 316, 1979.

Richardson U.I., Tashijan A.H. Jr., Levine L. Establishment of a clonal strain of hepatoma cells which secrete albumin.
J. Cell Biol. 40: 236, 1969.

Rosenbaum J.L., Kramer M.S., Raja R.M. Amberlite hemoperfusion in the treatment of acute drug intoxication.
Int. J. Artif. Org. 2: 316, 1979.

Rossi V., Malinverni A., Callegaro L. Immobilization of arginase on hollow fiber hemodialyzer.
Int. J. Artif. Org. 4: 102, 1981.

Schlansky R., Dettoratius R.J., Pinkus T., Tung K.S.K. Plasmapheresis in systemic lupus erythematosus. A cautionary note.
Arthritis Rheum, 24: 49, 1981.

Shinoda A., Kitada H., Suzuki S., Kurikara S., Saito Y., Yuri T., and Ishikawa I. Accessible plasma exchange using membrane filter. A successfully treated case of TTP with repeated plasma exchanges.
Artif. Organs, 5:3, 249, 1981.

Sieberth H.G. The elimination of defined substances from the blood and from separated plasma. In Plasma Exchange - Plasmapheresis - Plasmaseparation. International Symposium in Cologne, 6-7 June 1980.
H.G. Sieberth ed. Stuttgart, New York, (1980) p. 29.

Schmer G., Newman N.L., Rastelli L., Dennis M.B. Glutaraldehyde treated xenocell: a specific adsorbent for complement factors.
ASAIO 10: 57 (abstract), 1981.

Schmer G., Rastelli., Newman M.L., Dennis M.B., Holeenberg J.S. The bio-artificial organ.
Int. J. Artif. Org. 4: 96, 1981.

Schmer G., Krueger C.M., Cole J.J. Gel-bound released cell membranes: A new type of semi-artificial organs.
Trans. Am. Soc. Artif. Organs 23: 667, 1977.

Sedlacek H.H. Pathophysiological aspects of immune complex diseases. Part. 1 - Interaction with plasma enzyme systems, cell membranes and the immune response.
Klin. Wochenschr. 58: 543, 1980.

Senekjian H.O., Knight T.F., Weisman E.J. The spectrum of renal diseases associated with anti-basement membrane antibodies.
Arch. Intern. Med. 140: 79, 1980.

Shu C.D., Chang T.M.S. Tyrosinase immobilized artificial cells for detoxification in liver failure: II in vivo studies in fulminant hepatic failure rats.
Int. J. Art. Organs 4: 82, 1981.

Szpirer C., Szpirer J. A mouse hepatoma cell line which secrets serum proteins including albumin and α-fetoprotein.
Differentiation 4: 85, 1975.

Talpos G., Horrocks M., White J.M., Cotton L.T. Plasmapheresis in Raynaud's disease.
Lancet I 416, 1978.

Terman D.S. Tumoricidal responses in spontaneous canine neoplasms after extracorporeal perfusion over immobilized protein A.
Fed. Proc. Exp. Biol. 42: 45, 1981.

Terman D.S., Buffaloe G., Mattioli C., Cook G., Tillquist R., Sullivan M., Agus J.C. Extracorporeal immunoadsorption: initial experience in human systemic lupus erythematosus. Lancet II, 824, 1979.

Weiner H.L., and Dawson D.M. Plasmapheresis in multiple sclerosis: Preliminary study. Neurology, 30: 1029, 1980.

Weston M.J., Horak W., Gazzard B.G., Murray-Lyon I.M., Williams R. Bile acid removal from patients with liver diseases: model of artificial liver excretion. In Advances in Bile Acid Research. Matern S., Hackenschmidt J., Back P., Gerak W. eds. Stuttgart - New York: F.K. Schattener, 1975, p. 233.

Wieckowicz M. Single donor platelet transfusion: scientific, legal and ethical considerations. Transfusion 16: 193, 1976.

Winchester J.F., Gelfand M.C., Knepshield et al. Present and future uses of hemoperfusion with sorbents. Artif. Organs 2: 353, 1978.

World Healt Organization: The role of immune complexes in diseases. Technical Report Series 606, Geneve 5, 1977.

PATENTS

A survey of the patent situation on the title subject has been carried out by taking advantage of computer stored informations (Orbit IV) using as key word "hemodialysis" and "plasma treatment"

In order to identify the patent distribution these have been divided amongst Europe, U.S.A. and Japan.

Hemodialysis

EUROPE

Firm or author: Abadie A.

Title Prepn. of water for haemodialysis for e.g. renal haemodialysis by fixing acetate ions on exchange resin for water insol. ions and passing water over resin.

Priority FR-032009

Firm or author: ABG-SEMCA SA

Title Haemodialysis and blood ultrafiltration- ensuring precise flows and eliminating the risk of contamination.

Priority FR-014583

Firm or author: AGENCE NAT VALORISATION

Title Fluid agitation by applying controlled pressure waves to fluid in contact with elastic surface, facilitating heat or mass transfer. Haemodialysis.

Priority FR-000124

Firm or author: AKZO NV

Title Dialyser units, esp. for haemodialysis have bundles of hollow membrane fibres sealed into end sections with a polyurethane sealing compsn.

Priority DT-925172

Firm or author: AKZO NV

Title Dialysis membrane comprising thin walled hollow cellulose fibre- extruded from cuprammonium soln. of cellulose, used in haemodialysis.

Priority BE-879422

Firm or author: AKZO NV

Title Dialysis membrane comprising hollow cellulose fibre- with improved exchange surface in wavy form, mfd. from cuprammonium soln. of cellulose.

Priority BE-879110

Firm or author: AKZO NV

Title Dialysis membrane comprising hollow cellulose fibres- connected in parallel to fibres axis extruded from cuprammonium soln. of cellulose

Priority DT-906576

Firm or author: AKZO NV

Title Polyurethane coating compsns.- esp.for coating members for selective dialysers, e.g. for haemodialysis.

Priority DT-907501

Firm or author: AKZO NV

Title Dialysis membrane for haemodialysis- based on regenerated cellulose contg. adsorbents.

Priority DT-705734

Firm or author: AMERICAN HOSPITAL SUPPLY

Title Haemodialysis soln.- contg sorbitol and calcium ions.

Priority FR- 015621

Firm or author: APP ARTIFICIAL & TR

Title Haemodialysis appts. with dialysate tanks- each having concentrate inlet and outlet, metering pump and high and low level sensors for metering.

Priority GB-045266

Firm or author: AVON MEDICALS LTD

Title Fistula needle for haemodialysis- with outer plastics tube spaced around metal needle but fitting tightly near tip.

Priority GB-034116

Firm or author: BAYER AG

Title Dry-spinning hydrophilic hollow fibres from hydrophobic polymer- esp. acrylonitrile! polymer, using spinning dope having high solids and non-solvent conc.

Priority DT-804376

Firm or author: BEELEN R.

Title Precise meter system for ultrafiltration unit- for haemodialysis installation, has filter membrane and sampling circuit pump for single-pass flow.

Priority BE-834361

Firm or author: BEELEN R.

Title Haemodialysis needle- has hollow body divided in two for whole length.

Priority BE-834211

Firm or author: BELLCO SPA

Title Removing phosphates from haemodialysis liq.- by treatment with calcinated silica alumina mixts.

Priority IT-022320

Firm or author: BELLCO SPA

Title Removing urea from haemodialysis liquids- by treatment with oxidised starch

Priority IT-022319

Firm or author: BELLCO SPA

Title Removing ammonia from haemodialysis liq.- by treating with polyaldehyde, esp oxidised starch.

Priority IT-003409

Firm or author: BRET C D

Title Controlling ultrafiltration rate in haemodialysis- by controllable synchronous inlet and outlet pumps circulating dialysate through dialyser with pumped tapping off of ultrafiltrate.

Priority FR-002440

Firm or author: BONOMINI V

Title Portable haemodialysis appts.- has blood circuit and circuit for ultrafiltrate and dialysis liq.

Priority IT-003415

Firm or author: CAVAZZA C

Title Treating chronic uremia with acyl-carnitine- to prevent haemodialysis side-effects, e.g. asthenia.

Priority BE-876262

Firm or author: CAVAZZA C

Title Use of carnitine to prevent myocardiopathy- in patients with chronic uraemia undergoing haemodialysis.

Priority IT-049355

Firm or author:CENT D'HEMODIALYSE

Title Fully automatic washing and sterilizing of haemodialyser for reuse- greatly increases utilisation of scarce equipment without skilled operator.

Priority FR-042796

Firm or author: DANSKE SUKKERFAB A/S

Title Membrane support plate for haemodialysis stack-having integral flaps fold-able to secure the membrane and form blood flow conduits.

Priority DK-003642

Firm or author: DANSKE SUKKERFAB A/S

Title Haemodializer membrane support- improved flow path reduces membrane area and treatment time

Priority DK-003641

Firm or author: FRAUMHOFER-GES FORD ANGE

Title Automatic regulator for haemodialysis appts.- with continuous extraction of water from patients during dialysis.

Priority DT-644062

Firm or author: FRESENIUS CHEM PHAR

Title Ultrafiltration control appts. for haemodialysis treatment- has automatic timer for connecting storage containers for dialysis liq. to circulatory system in timed sequence.

Priority DT-734561

Firm or author: FRESENIUS E CHEM

Title Pumping system for haemodialysis appts.- controls rate of dialysis accurately adjustable.

Priority DT-544258

Firm or author: FRESENIUS E CHEM

Title Puncture needle for artificial kidney haemodialysis- with eliptical needle tip for smaller incision wound.

Priority DT-452223

Firm or author: HOECHST AG

Title Viscose haemodialysis membranes-highly oriented equally in both directions, have improved permeability properties.

Priority DT-736569

Firm or author: HOECHST AG

Title Selective permeability hetero-porous polyamide films- useful in haemodialysis, esp. of blood in the treatment of kidney disease.

Priority DT-704600

Firm or author:HOSPAL SA

Title Haemodialyser incorporating flattened tubular semipermeable membrane- has membrane wound spirally around mandrel composed of two similar longitudinal elements joined together, minimising complexity and cost.

Priority IT-069802

Firm or author: INST NAT SANTE RECH MED

Title Haemodialysis with automatic control- by continuous monitor of body wt. and blood pressure.

Priority FR-023423

Firm or author: KLAUSCHENZ & PERROT

Title Blood spillage indication system during haemodialysis- introduces flushing liq. tangentially into measuring chamber to give centrifugal effect.

Priority DT-611383

Firm or author: LUCAS IND LTD

Title Haemodialysis mach. blood return cut-off- is effected by tube grippers actuated in response to air bubble.

Priority GB-010921

Firm or author: LUCAS IND LTD

Title Bubble detector for haemodialysis mach.- comprises a photocell unit monitoring a fluid flow tube.

Priority GB-010920

Firm or author: MEDICAL DEVELOPMENT

Title Industrial scale production of multiple bed haemodialysis units- by winding on a drum alternate layers of support and tubular membrane.

Priority BE-859000

Firm or author: NATIONAL RESEARCH DEVELOP

Title Plate dialysers esp. haemodialysers.

Priority GB-031244

Firm or author: ORGANON TEKNIKA

Title Selective diffusion separator- using semipermeable membranes particularly for haemodialysis.

Priority NL-002881

Firm or author: RHONE-POULENC IND

Title Artificial kidney providing haemodialysis and two way ultrafiltration- by establishing press. difference between blood and dialysis liq.

Priority FR-014007

Firm or author: RHONE-POULENC IND

Title Insert for membrane exchange or sepn. appts.- with ribs supporting membrane and allowing circulation, useful in haemodialysis, etc.

Priority FR-034610

Firm or author: RHONE-POULENC SA

Title Haemodialysis blood circuit- has pipes, pump and accessories forming variable volume blood chamber.

Priority FR-033982

Firm or author: RHONE-POULEC SA

Title Artificial haemodialysis kidney- with constant volume closed vessel in form of a loop which can be isolated to form a closed circuit.

Priority FR-027582

Firm or author: RHONE-POULENC SA

Title Dialysis liq. generator- for suppling dialysis liq. to haemodialysers.

Priority FR-000247

Firm or author: RHONE-POULENC IND

Title Condensation prod. of hexa:methylene di:iso-cyanate and acrylate- useful in bonding hol-low fibres e.g. for haemodialysis.

Priority FR-024841

Firm or author: SCHILLING B

Title Sterilisable membranes for haemodialysis-comprising uniformly sized and spaced holes in metal sheet.

Priority DT-559332

Firm or author: SIREN M

title Treatment of dialysis membrane units- with a reagent which dissolves out cadmium.

Priority SW-002005

Firm or author: SIREN M

Title Semipermeable cuprammonium regenerated cellu-lose membrane prodn.- including cleaning sta-ges to remove cadmium.

Priority SW-002004

Firm or author: SISTER SPA

Title Aero-embolism preventer for hydraulic circuits-has float housed in chamber engaging inner walls to form air-tight seal between chamber and outlet.

Priority IT-027072

Firm or author: SMITHS IND LTD

Title Bubble-traps and liquid-supply equipment for haemodialysis- comprising collection chamber with inlets disposed above normal blood level.

Priority GB-008953

Firm or author: SODIP

Title Extracorporeal blood purificn.- by simultaneous

haemodialysis and haemo-filtration with incorporated flow equilibration.

Priority FR-031918

Firm or author: SORIN RIC BIOMED

Title Recovery of electrolytic solutions for haemodialysis- with control by automatic regulation of diluent water flow rate.

Priority IT-069835

Firm or author: TERSTEEGEN B

Title Extracorporeal haemodialysis duplex channel catheter- having inner and outer tubes arranged to provide for uniform outflow of blood through annular duct between tubes.

Priority DT-703087

Firm or author: TERSTEEGEN B

Title Twin channel catheter for haemodialysis- has concentric channels and outer tube is cut away to form sharp edge.

Priority DT-613281

Firm or author: VDO A SCHINDLING A G

Title Press. indicator for haemodialysis instrument- has cylindrical housing with connecting pipe at one end and cover at other end.

Priority DT-320327

Firm or author: VERDER-VLEUTEN BV

Title Continuous automated prodn. of haemodialyser fluid- concentrate and water continuously metered into vessel with composition controlled by conductivity cells.

Priority NL-010758

Firm or author: VLAHO M

Title Air embolism prevention in haemodialysis- has metal indicator float coated with teflon.

Priority DT-310931

U.S.A.

Firm or author: ABCOR INC

Title Semipermeable membrane for hemodialysis or desalination-has polyethylene imine grafts on e.g. cellulose or polyamides.

Priority US-195881

Firm or author: AMER HOSPITAL SUPPL CORP

Title Semipermeable membrane mass transfer appts.- -has membrane folded in accordion pleats whose creases are embedded in plastics at their ends.

Priority US-779576

Firm or author: BARD C R INC

Title Polyether-polycarbonate copolymer hemodialysis membrane- with improved diffusion permeability and ultrafiltration speed.

Priority US-672354

Firm or author: BARD C R INC

Title Hydrophilic polycarbonate hemodialysis membranes- which give high rates of filtration and improved condition of patient during treatment.

Priority US-668556

Firm or author: BAXTER LAB

Title Housing for a hemodialysis unit- including a cover which allows the transmembrane pressure to be controlled.

Priority US-068294

Firm or author: BIGI L

Title Phosphate ion removal from dialysing liquids in hemodialysis- by contact with activated mixt. of alumina and silica.

Priority US-685024

Firm or author: BOWMAN D B

Title Hemodialysis system including water and

dialysate pumps- each comprising a rotable reciprocable piston linked by reduction gearing.

Priority US-479998

Firm or author: CALIFORNIA INST TECHN

Title Hemodialysis system for selective removal of urea- by dialysis through a cationic polymeric membrane into a decomposition chamber.

Priority US-772434

Firm or author: COBE LABS INC

Title Rotatable mount for hemodialyser- has latching mechanism for securing dialyser in upright and inverted positions.

Priority US-844144

Firm or author: COBE LAB INC

Title Mfr. of fluid flow transfer appts.- uses injection of potting material to ensure firm anchorage of membrane tips.

Priority US-784364

Firm or author: COBE LAB INC

Title Pleated membrane fluid flow transfer appts.- has outer sealing compartements for potting membrane flaps; used for blood hemodialysis, etc.

Priority US-906064

Firm or author: CORDIS DOW CORP

Title Automatic regulation of hemodialysis- at preselected ultrafiltration speed using two double chambered cylinders feeding and wasting alternately.

Priority US-958329

Firm or author: CORDIS DOW CORP

Title Continuous formation and supply of hemodialysis

soln.- with partial replacement of sodium acetate by sodium bi:carbonate.

Priority US-927322

Firm or author: COSENTINO L C

Title Hemodialysis ultrafiltration circuit- which permits ultrafiltration rate to be controlled during hemodialysis.

Priority US-622755

Firm or author: DOW CHEM CO

Title Hemodialysis with highly permeable membranes- with control to prevent high ultrafiltration rates or reverse ultrafiltration.

Priority US-257450

Firm or author: EXXON & ENG CO

Title Hemodialysis device for removal of urea and other toxins from blood- utilising liquid membrane capsules contg. citric acid.

Priority US-005353

Firm or author: GALEN LAB INC

Title Semipermeable membrane, particularly for hemodialysis folded in form of a stackwithin a housing, has edges sealed in solidifiable liq.

Priority US-373160

Firm or author: GENERAL ELECTRIC CO

Title Dialysis stack for hemodialysis- with flexible membrane supports permitting blood passage expansion with increasing pressure.

Priority US-051829

Firm or author: HOECHST AG

Title Peristaltic pump for a hemodialysis unit- comprising a silicone rubber diaphragm tube and a rotary pump head with rollers.

Priority US-888858

Firm or author: HOECHST AG

Title Blood leak detection in hemodialysis system- by measuring variations in reflecting light received by photodetector on same side of dialysate flow-stream as transmitter.

Priority US-888859

Firm or author: HOLMAN D G

Title Umbillical cord pre-shaping for use as blood--vessel implants- takes place by placing on mandrel, extracting water, fixing with aldehyde soln. and pref. roughening.

Priority US-872606

Firm or author: HUTCHINSON J L

Title Antithrombogenic hemodialysis membranes- comprising partially decarboxylated cellulose.

Priority US-667539

Firm or author: IBM CORP

Title Automated hemodialysis treatment system- controls ultrafiltration rate to preset value and measures rate and ultrafiltrate removed.

Priority US-749585

Firm or author: LAVENDER A R

Title Mass transfer device for blood oxygenation, dialysis etc.- has alternating plates and membranes with baffles providing uniform fluid distribution to and from each plate.

Priority US-733445

Firm or author:MAHURKAR S D

Title Double lumen hemodialysis catheter- with lumen ends spaced and bevelled to prevent flows mixing.

Priority US-812901

Firm or author: MEDICAL INC

Title Hemodialyser incorporating semi-permeable membrane in box- using membrane with predetermined moisture content, maintained constant to utilisation time.

Priority US-672853

Firm or author: MEDICAL DEVICE LAB

Title Single hypodermic puncture for extn. and return blood flow- esp. for hemodialysis or oxigenation of blood.

Priority US-620600

Firm or author:NEWHART E E

Title Integral artificial kidney unit- comprises a plastic dyalisate chamber enclosing plastic perfusion units permeable to waste excreta in blood.

Priority US-799501

Firm or author: NEWHART E E

Title Ambulatory self-contained hemodialysis unit- has perfusion unit, dialysate reservor and pump actuated by patient generated pulses.

Priority US-281183

Firm or author: PINKERTON H

Title Proportioning fluids in hemodialysis systems- using hydraulic circuit having double-acting piston and cylinder unit with differing swept vol.

Priority US-687133

Firm or author: PUROPORE INC

Title Dense hollow fibre membrane for hemodialysis- formed by dry spinning soln. of cellulose acetate and oligosaccharide ester.

Priority US-950664

Firm or author: RAULERSON J D

Title Dual purpose catheter for hemodialysis- has adapter with two fluid ducts and concentric cannula elements.

Priority US-652288

Firm or author: RENAL SYSTEMS INC

Title Blending hemodialysate from multiple fluid concentrate- by multichamber metering pump with valves controlled by piston position.

Priority US-804505

Firm or author: RENAL SYSTEMS INC

Title Blood air leak detector for hemodialysis etc- has optical sensor adjacent tube monitoring flow for bubbles.

Priority US-524329

Firm or author: SANDOZ SA

Title Artificial kidney hemodialysis membrane element- comprising flat open frame carrying membrane tube bundle.

Priority US-456695

Firm or author: SANDOZ AG

Title Monitor for hemodialysis plant- gives alarm and pump stop signal when blood withdrawal and return cycle is too long.

Priority US-393101

Firm or author: TEXAS MED PROD INC

Title Bifurcated tubing connector for hemodialysis- comprises three modular parts hollow body, contoured cover and tube coupling.

Priority US-555749

Firm or author: THOMPSON L E

Title Blood leak detector for hemodialysis systems- has screen preventing dialysate bubbles from entering detecting light beam.

Priority US-723924

Firm or author: TRI-FLO RES LAB LTD

Title Dialyser using hypertonic and hypotonic solns.- giving good dialysis rate in parallel plate hemodialyser.

Priority US-461461

Firm or author: UNION CARBIDE CORP

Title Portable hemodialysis unit- having integral adsorber for purifying dialysis liquor.

Priority US-636062

Firm or author: UNIVERSITY OF UTAH

Title Cellulose hemodialysis membrane cast from cupriethylene- diamine hydroxide solns.

Priority US-020029

Firm or author: US SEC OF AGRICULTURE

Title Polyether polycarbonate copolymer membranes for hemodialysis- having improved permeability to solutes in middle molecule range.

Priority US-636062

Firm or author: US SEC OF HEALTH

Title Polyether-polycarbonate block copolymer prodn.- from polyether glycol cpd., bisphenol=A, pyridine and phosgene, used in forming hemodialysis membranes.

Priority US-873168

Firm or author: USA SEC of Health

Title Polyvinyl pyrrolidone-cellulose acetate hemodialysis membranes- permeable to inulin but not albumin.

Priority US-256512

Firm or author: US SEC HEALTH

Title Non-thrombogenic hemodialysis hollow fibre

membranes- used in artificial kidney and prepd from mixt. of acrylonitrile/vinyl acetate and acrylonitrile/vinyl pyridine copolymers.

Priority US-102132

Firm or author: US SEC OF HEALTH

Title Non-thrombogenic hemodialysis flat membranes- made from quaternised membrane of vinyl pyridine-contg polymer useful in artificial kidneys.

Priority US-102092

Firm or author: US DEPT ENERGY

Title Disposable hemodialyser with flattened membranes tubes- in which blood passes successively over two groups of tubes.

Priority US-822861

Firm or author: US GOVERNMENT

Title Polyether-polycarbonate block copolymer films- esp for hemodialysis made by casting from soln.

Priority US-454949

Firm or author: US GOVERNMENT

Title Polycarbonate membrane for hemodialysis- by forming polycarbonate-polyether-solvent-cosolvent sheet, partly driyng and immersing in water.

Priority US-454939

Firm or author: VITAL ASSISTS INC

Title Blood port assembly for hemodialysis- with positive positionining and sealing.

Priority US-243016

Firm or author: VITAL ASSIST INC

Title Membrane support plate for hemodialysis stacks- including a removable veneer provided with rows of membrane supporting wedges

Priority US-242994

Firm or author: VITAL ASSISTS INC

Title Hemodialyser- with dialysate flowing transversely accross pleated membrane having pleats separated by spacers.

Priority US-106184

JAPAN

Firm or author: ASAHI MEDICAL CO

Title Hollow-fibre dialysis membranes- of polyether-polycarbonate block copolymers with improved permeability and mechanical properties.

Priority JA-004311

Firm or author: ASAHI MEDICAL CO

Title Hemodialyser comprising hollow fibres- which are loosely bundled and pass diagonally across dialysate vessel to give improved performance.

Priority JA-U48873

Firm or author: KURARAY KK

Title Ethylene!-vinyl! alcohol copolymer hollow fibre membrane- has circular cross section and three-layer structure contg. two bonded particle layers.

Priority JA-053031

Firm or author: KURARAY KK

Title Asymmetric semipermeable membranes- made from mixts. of ethylene!-vinyl! alcohol copolymers with different ethylene! contents.

Priority JA-108251

Firm or author: TAKEDA CHEMICAL IND KK

Title Closed hemodialysis circuits- developing required pressure in auxiliary pipe between dialysate source and pump outside closed loop.

Priority JA-069343

Firm or author: TAKEDA CHEMICAL INDS LTD

Title Artificial kidney hemodialyser- has semipermeable material separating chambers, with adsorbing material for dialysate.

Firm or author: TORAY IND INC

Title Semi-permeable pref hemodialysis hydrogel membrane- prepd from iso-tactic and syndiotactic polymethyl methacrylate mixture sol by gelling and solvent displacement.

Priority JA-018879

Plasma Treatment

EUROPE

Firm or author: COMMISS ENERGIE ATOMIQUE

Title Extn. and purification of thyroxine binding globulin- from protein fraction of human plasma by chromathography.

Priority FR-036668

Firm or author: IMMUNO CHEM MED AG

Title Prodn. of purified plasma protein- by stepwise enrichment in presence of fast-reacting anti-thrombin.

Priority OE-002940

Firm or author: KABI AB

Title Purification of heparin used in thrombosis treatment- by adsorption on a matrix to which a plasma protein is fixed.

Priority SW-003040

Firm or author: LAEVOSAN-GES MBH

Title Plasma expander hydroxyethyl-starch purification- by extracting with solvent e.g. DMF to separate from salts.

Priority OE-002489

Firm or author: NORDISK INSULINLAB

Title Recovering purified albumin from human blood plasma- using polyethylene glycol in fractional precipitation process.

Priority DK-000258

Firm or author: PHARMACIA FINE CHEM

Title Albumin ion-exchange isolation from plasma products- by treating partially purified plasma with an anion-exchanger and a cation--exchanger.

Priority SW-011295

Firm or author: PLIS B

Title Purification of hyperimmune horse plasma.

Priority FR-095286

Firm or author: RECH HEMATOLOGISQUES

Title Concn. and purification of anti:haemophilia factor- by extraction of a cryogenic ppte. from plasma with an aq. medium and cooling to ppte. fibrinogen.

Priority DT-636757

Firm or author: RUDOLPH W

Title Hepatitis antigen test serum prodn.- by injecting a horse with purified australia positive plasma.

Priority DL-166397

Firm or author: UK ATOMIC ENERGY

Title Purification of factor VIII in aq. soln. esp. Blood plasma- by continuous flow electrophoresis.

Priority GB-047933

Firm or author: WELLCOME FOUNDATION LTD

Title Serum or plasma purification for immunoglobulin M detection- by contacting with immobilised immunoglobulin G and staphylococcal protein A

Priority GB-05008

Firm or author: ZIMMER AG PLANUNG UND BAU

Title Polyvinylpyrrolidone purification- by extn with liquid halohydrocarbon, for blood plasma substitute, tablet binder etc.

Priority DT-V32022

U.S.A.

Firm or author: ARMOUR PHARM CO

Title Purified plasma albumin of unmodified characteristics- is obtained by passing plasma fraction through ion exchange resins at ph below and then above albumin isoelectic point.

Priority US-014837

Firm or author: ARMOUR PHARM CO

Title Plasminogen purifcn. from human or non-human mammalian plasma- by affinity chromatography using sepharose 1-lysine with high ionic strength buffer solns.

Priority US-440206

Firm or author: BIOTEST SERUM INST GMBH

Title Hepatitis-safe prods. from citrate-stabilised plasma- by treating with ion exchange resins in the prepn. of anti:haemophilic globulin A, prothrombin complex, fibrinogen and a serum protein.

Priority US-875489

Firm or author: CUTTER LABS

Title Hydrolase purified from human plasma- which can activate and degrade Factor VIII, activate Factor V, and inhibit platelet aggregation.

Priority US-054127

Firm or author: JURIDICAL FOUNDATIO

Title Purificn. of hepatitis B surface antigen from blood plasma or serum- by passage through anion then cation exchanger.

Priority US-946733

Firm or author: MINNESOTA UNIVERSITY

Title Isolation and purification of gamma-globulin and albumin- by treating blood plasma with silica then with ion exchange.

Priority US-829565

Firm or author: MINNESOTA UNIVERSITY

Title Plasma purified by contact with fumed colloidal silica- for perfusing transplant kidneys and for treating haemorrhagic shock.

Priority US-570569

Firm or author: SHANBROM E

Title Conc. and purifcn. of Factor VIII from plasma- using selective pptn. of low ionic strength soln. at low temp. to remove fibrinogen and its denaturated and degradaded prods.

Priority US-899235

Firm or author: SHANBRON E INC

Title Conc, and purificn. of plasma antihaemophilic factor- by cryoprecipitation, extn. into water cooling to ppte. fibrinogen and lyophilising.

Priority US-586948

Firm or author: UPJOHN CO

Title Gamma-globulin purification- by contact with solid plasma protein for specific removal of undesirable antibodies only.

Priority US-165697

Firm or author: UPJOHN CO

Title Purification of gamma-globulin from serum- or plasma.

Priority US-016225

Firm or author: WILSON W L

Title Purified antitrombin III isolation from plasma- by adsorption on aluminium hydroxide gel and precipitation of albumins and globulins with polyoxyalkylene cpds.

Priority US-694167

JAPAN

Firm or author: ASAHI CHEMICAL IND KK

Title Medical purifier for removal of DNA and complexes from blood or plasma- comprises hydrophilic solid, polysaccharide and glass particles with adsorbent layer on the surface comprising an ion exchanger.

Priority JA-035069

Firm or author: ASAHI CHEMICAL IND KK

Title Device for purificn. of blood by removal of waste and uebris- comprising a plasma sepg. membrane, a purifier and a mixer.

Priority JA-033562

Firm or author: GREEN CROSS CORP

Title Cholinesterase prodn. from human blood plasma- by selective pptn. and extn. using polyethylene glycol!, anion exchange resin, ammonium sulphate, and sodium sulphate.

Priority JA-005302

Firm or author: GREEN CROSS CORP

Title Antihaemophilic globulin A isolation from plasma- by treatment with anion exchanger.

Priority JA-039894

Firm or author: GREEN CROSS CORP

Title High-purity human serum haptoglobin solns- prepd by anion-exchanger treatment of pptd. plasma globulin fractions.

Priority JA-128606

Firm or author: KAGAKU OYOBI KESSEI

Title Type C hepatitis virus antigen- obtd. by gel filtration, ion-exchange chromatography and centrifugation of plasma or serum of non-A, non-B hepatitis.

Priority JA-030332

Firm or author: KAGAKU OYOBI KESSEI

Title Purificn. of hepatitis B surface antigen from plasma and serum- in fractions passing freely through columns of anion and cation exchanger.

Priority JA-036555

Firm or author: TOKUYAMA SODA KK

Title Imparting selectivity to cation exchange membrane- by effecting plasma polymerisation in presence of nitrogen cpd. to form nitrogen-contg. polymer layer on membrane.

Priority JA-030477

POSTSCRIPT

Forecasting and Assessment in the Field of Science and Technology.

The Council of Ministers of the European Communities decided in 1978 to initiate a five year experimental programme 'Forecasting and Assessment in the Field of Science and Technology (FAST)', which was implemented in 1979.

The main aim of FAST is to contribute to the definition of long-term community research and development objectives and priorities and thus to the formulation of a coherent science and technology policy in the long-term.

To this end, the programme has to highlight prospects, problems and potential conflicts likely to affect the long-term development of the community with an orientation towards defining alternative courses of community research and development action to help or solve or achieve them or to render concrete those possibilities.

The programme has also to encourage the establishment of an ad hoc system of collaboration in the form of networks, as informal and flexible as possible, between community centres specialising in forecasting and assessment in the field of science and technology.

FAST is not intended to predict the future but rather to study the possible sources of alternative developments and hence to throw light on possible and desirable options for R&D policy. A central tenet of the programme is that possible futures are not a matter of chance: they will be as our societies determine them.

Within this mandate three sub-programmes reflecting problem areas of three different time horizons have been defined:

1. Work and employment
2. 'Information-Society'
3. 'Bio-Society'

50 European research teams have been working for FAST on 30 research projects:

Work and employment
- prospects for the European chemical industry
- prospects for the construction industry
- the future of repair activities
- the development of the environmental industry
- the future of employment in the services
- regional prospects of employment in Europe
- biomass, regions and employment
- attitudes towards work
- social innovations in the 80's
- productivity and progress
- small enterprises, technical change and employment

Information society
- microelectronics innovations in the context of the international division of labour
- job creation potential of the information technologies
- long-term options and forecasts for transport in Europe
- representation and sharing of power in an information society
- the impact of information technologies on the way of life: work, leisure, transport and communications
- distributions of benefits and risks associated with microelectronics applications
- man-machine relations: dangers and remedies

Biosociety
- a community strategy for European biotechnology
- biotechnologies in the production of chemical feedstocks and derived products
- proteins: probable impacts and development strategies for biotechnology in European agro-food systems

- community strategy for biotechnology: analysis of scientific disciplines germane to biotechnology
- information technologies in the development of biotechnology (bio-informatics)
- manpower and training implications of the expansion of biotechnology-based industries
- social dimensions of biotechnologies, social and political choices that may be created by progress in biotechnologies
- proteins: implications of biotechnologies for developing countries and international trade
- implications for the third world of biotechnology
- technological forecasts of downstream processing in biotechnology
- detoxification as therapeutic techniques, problems and prospects
- environmental biotechnology: future prospects